Managing Yourself
On and Off The Ward

Michael Walton
PhD, MA, MSc, BA, FIPD, AFBPsS, C.Psychol

Blackwell
Science

© 1995 by
Blackwell Science Ltd
Editorial Offices:
Osney Mead, Oxford OX2 0EL
25 John Street, London WC1N 2BL
23 Ainslie Place, Edinburgh EH3 6AJ
238 Main Street, Cambridge,
  Massachusetts 02142, USA
54 University Street, Carlton,
  Victoria 3053, Australia

Other Editorial Offices:
Arnette Blackwell SA
  1, rue de Lille, 75007 Paris
  France

Blackwell Wissenschafts-Verlag GmbH
  Kurfürstendamm 57
  10707 Berlin, Germany

Feldgasse 13, A-1238 Wien
Austria

First published 1995

Set by DP Photosetting, Aylesbury, Bucks
Printed and bound in Great Britain by
Hartnolls Ltd, Bodmin, Cornwall

DISTRIBUTORS

Marston Book Services Ltd
PO Box 87
Oxford OX2 0DT
(*Orders:* Tel: 01865 791155
         Fax: 01865 791927
         Telex: 837515)

North America
  Blackwell Science, Inc.
  238 Main Street
  Cambridge, MA 02142
  (*Orders:* Tel: 800 215-1000
           617 876-7000
           Fax: 617 492-5263)

Australia
  Blackwell Science Pty Ltd
  54 University Street
  Carlton, Victoria 3053
  (*Orders:* Tel: 03 347-0300
           Fax: 03 349-3016)

A catalogue record for this book is available
from the British Library

ISBN 0-632-03447-5

Library of Congress
Cataloging in Publication Data
Walton, Michael, PhD.
    Managing yourself on and off the ward/
    Michael Walton.
       p. cm.
    Includes bibliographical references and
index.
    ISBN 0-632-03447-5
    1. Nursing–Practice.   2. Nursing–
Psychological aspects.
    3. Organizational behavior.
    4. Organizational change.
    5. Interpersonal relations.
    6. Nursing–Practice–Great Britain.
    I. Title.
    RT86.7.W35   1995
    362.1'73'068–dc20   95-1076
                                            CIP

This book is dedicated to

Frances Mary Walton – nearly lost

and

Kenneth Wagner Tobias – recently found

Contents

PART THREE: INTERACTIONS, INFLUENCE AND INTERFERENCE

Foreword

Yvonne Moores
*Chief Nursing Officer and Director of Nursing
Department of Health*

I am pleased to write the Foreword for Michael Walton's interesting and stimulating exploration of personal effectiveness through management of yourself as a nurse.

I believe that personal effectiveness is attained through, amongst other qualities, the acquisition of specific attributes and the maximizing of opportunities as these present. Calling on the wisdom and experiences of the people available to you also serve to lay the foundation necessary for the development of the individual nurse. You can never tell which event, personal or professional, will be the one that unexpectedly provides the opportunity for you to demonstrate effectiveness. The key is having the necessary resources to respond in an effective way as such occurrences become a proving ground for the individual nurse.

Nurses wherever or with whomever they work will identify with this, and will readily recall people and situations which could be described as character forming and where personal effectiveness was enhanced as a result of their involvement.

Dr Walton's book will help you understand how similar your colleagues, patients, managers and you are in the way you think, feel and act. You will realize that large organizations or groups of people behave in particular ways. Understanding these matters will enable you to gear your actions, attitudes and knowledge to be as effective as you can when dealing with patients, colleagues, or other people. Although the benefits derived through knowledge gained should enhance your effectiveness and impact in a positive way with those with whom you interact.

Preface

Welcome. I hope you will find this book to be both practical and enjoyable to use. It is focused on *you* and your relationships at work – but you can apply the ideas to all aspects of your life because it offers a variety of ways to re-examine what is going on around you.

The book's specific purpose is to support you in what you are doing, and to help you become a more effective and purposeful nurse in whatever roles you choose throughout your career. You do not have to aspire to being a top nurse to find this book of value but you do have to have an interest in being more effective and perceptive.

In my experience books about management are often boring and far removed from the day-to-day issues, anxieties and concerns of work, and consequently they just aren't used and are solemnly stashed away in the loft or left around to impress others. I hope no such fate awaits this book. I hope it will become dog-eared and well-used – wrinkled even – and that you will find it a great help in alerting (and reminding) you about what may be going on (in and around you) as you go about your work. I hope it becomes a friend and a companion, that you refer to it often, and that it will help you time and time again, even though it doesn't try to cover everything and even though you could probably have written some parts of it better than I have.

I have not overloaded the book with too many theories, but have stayed with notions you can use and develop further for yourself. You will find that I have frequently used diagrams to present the ideas. I realize that not everyone likes diagrams but they can often capture vividly and succinctly what is involved in a situation. In this way too the message can be presented more powerfully and with more impact. However, if you find they get on your nerves please look to see what I am getting at and then put my ideas into your own most helpful alternative format. My only wish is that you work through and consider the various points raised – how you do it is up to you!

There are also quite a few tables that need to be completed. Completing the various exercises makes the material come alive and it will help you in your practical work with patients, relatives and colleagues. Incidentally, do remember to make a note of the date when you complete the exercises, because going back over your earlier perspectives and ideas will help you keep track of how they have altered and developed over the years. Looking back in this way can be very constructive especially if you are coaching more junior colleagues.

Managing Yourself On and Off the Ward is a handbook rather than a learned text that has all the answers, and while it is deliberately non-academic I have drawn from a wide range of source material, some of which is academic. I hope you will wish to pursue in more detail some of the ideas I have drawn attention to and the reading lists at the end of most chapters are included to help you do this.

In undertaking your work there are few certainties about exactly how to handle the complexities of the interpersonal dynamics, tensions and stresses that are involved when people try to relate to and work with each other.

What you can do though is:

(1) try to clarify what is going on within yourself and with others;
(2) have a reservoir of relevant ideas and notions that help to throw more light on what you are experiencing; and then
(3) use these perspectives to decide how best to respond in the circumstances.

The book is designed to help you to tune into, come to terms with, and then act responsibly and ethically in relation to the ever-changing situations in which you find yourself. While there may not always be opportunities to exercise complete freedom in what you do – because of clinical, legal, professional or other restrictions – you can nevertheless be yourself in what you do and take strength from managing yourself with integrity.

Most of the book keeps the focus on *you* and, as you work through the book, you will be able to build up a clearer picture of what is important to you and to draw up more ideas about what makes you tick. As I noted earlier, do keep a record of your thoughts as you go through the book – you will find them interesting to look at in the years ahead because they will give you information about how you have changed over the intervening period.

This book is *not* focused on the clinical procedures you follow or have been taught, but on how you establish, maintain and develop the relationships you have with colleagues and patients; matters connected with interpersonal dynamics and relationships, and how they are influenced by the settings in which people come together to work.

Two areas of great significance which are often neglected are how the culture of the organization affects its operational effectiveness, and how members of staff bring not only their professional expertise and experience but also their personalities and individuality to their jobs.

Figure P.1 contrasts these two areas with two others (a concern for structure and an emphasis on roles, tasks and procedures) which are usually the focus of attention.

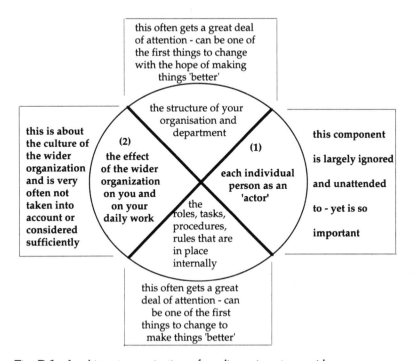

Fig. P.1 Looking at organizations: four dimensions to consider.

In this book the emphasis is on the two neglected areas of (1) you as *yourself* in a health care setting, and (2) the culture of organizations and how they seem to work (or not, as the case may be) and in turn affect your well-being and operational effectiveness.

This is also a book about *leadership* as well as *management*. Each of us is a leader irrespective of any formal job title we might hold and so I believe we can't escape from being a leader, a manager and a follower all at the same time. Therefore the more we understand about leadership, the better we will become at effectively handling such responsibilities. What I am suggesting is that we all have personal responsibility for exercising leadership of our thoughts and actions, and in addition to this we sometimes find we have similar formalized responsibilities at work and formal job titles to go with those responsibilities.

Why bother – what is it all about?

When you are under pressure or in trying circumstances you can easily lose sight of what is going on around you and of what you are trying to do. One way of keeping matters in perspective – and coping better with these pressures – is to build up your own set of 'ways of looking at things' that will help you to make sense of what is going on and where you stand within those situations. If you can do this you will have more insight and an opportunity to make better informed decisions about what to do rather than just reacting to alleviate the immediate difficulty.

Caring for others, who invariably are worried, dependent and vulnerable, carries with it both satisfaction and considerable professional and personal responsibility. When the pressure is on it can be all too easy to focus on the most immediate task (to the exclusion of everything else) and forget the wider caring work you are involved in. This carries with it a risk of metaphorically pushing the patient out of the way and of reducing them to objects which have to be dealt with in mechanical ways.

Even though the specific task of that moment *is* critical it is not 'task completion' alone which is likely to be the critical facet of your continuing contact with a patient, except of course in life threatening situations. At the core of the psychological well-being of the patient (which will influence their physical state) is the nature, tone and pattern of your human 'engagement' with them. In health care the interactive and qualitative aspects of care assume critical importance. I believe that it is also the same for you in relation to your colleagues, other professional carers, relatives, family, *et al.*

This book is worth bothering with because it aims to help you secure a focused, realistically based and positive sense of yourself and your relationship to others. I see this as determining to a very great extent the quality of the psychological care you are able to offer to others around you. If you feel bad about yourself you are less able to care fully for others. If you feel good about yourself and your capabilities you are more likely to take the daily bumps and bruises in your stride, and care for others more successfully. This book provides material to help you become a little clearer about who you are, what you are after and how to work more effectively with others.

Overview of the book

The book is organized into five parts and you will get most value from it if you initially flip through the whole thing to give you an overall sense of the flow, style and general pattern of the material, before dipping in at random as your needs and interests take you. The sequence I have followed is:

Part One   – The dynamics of the social world, the NHS, and some perspectives on organizations.

Part Two	– Thinking about yourself and what is important to you.
Part Three	– Working with others, handling differences, leadership and management.
Part Four	– Change management processes and the nurse as a facilitator of change.
Part Five	– Pulling it all together which offers some concluding thoughts and perspectives.

Part One sets the scene for the book. It starts by looking at the interactive aspects of your work as a person – with your own personal beliefs and views – when working with others; the social *dynamics* of your relationships. A brief overview of the main organizational changes to the NHS since its inception then provides a historical perspective for you to look again at current developments. Chapter 3 introduces ideas about organizations as much of your working life this will be the operational context within which you will work.

You are the main focus of this book and the views you have about yourself are considered in Part Two. How you view and value yourself, where you see yourself going, what matters to you and how this can alter over time are explored in some detail because of their critical importance for your professional practice and well-being.

Enhanced understanding of yourself is just as important as the recognition that each of us sees and makes sense of the social world around us in different ways. An appreciation of these differences is essential if you are to work effectively with others. If you are able to begin to understand how others view matters you are more likely to be able to build a better caring–treatment alliance. Yourself *with* others is the focus for Part Three.

In Part Four the emphasis moves to the dynamics of change. In spite of the many books and articles produced this remains a field of study that continues to baffle many people. I think this is partly because of an over emphasis on establishing the logic for a change – and hoping others will be swayed by this – and the relative neglect of non-rational factors that are triggered when 'change' is mentioned. Part Four also considers the role of the nurse as a promoter of 'change'.

Finally Part Five re-asserts the importance of self-knowledge and understanding, and a knowledge and understanding of organizational processes if you are to be fully effective at work.

Using the book

The material covered will complement, and possibly, challenge some of your current ideas and will provide a basis for you to review what you do *in practice*. You are asked to relate the ideas introduced to your own experiences and to reflect on what you do in practice. While this is valuable in itself, you can get even more from the material if you are able to compare your thoughts and experiences with colleagues. It can be reassuring to find that you have similar views and experiences and it can be instructive to note, and then to explore, where there are differences and why that might be.

So when you feel you can, and when it is practicable, consider working through some of the material with colleagues as a way of exploring more fully the ideas introduced, and as a way of building up mutually supportive relationships. I suggest it would be important to reach an agreement that such discussions remain confidential.

Many of the ideas in this book can also be used for group training sessions and could provide the core material for further exploration and development of individual skills and effective group working.

While focused towards nursing and health care settings, almost all of the ideas and perspectives presented in the book can be applied to your non-nursing worlds. You may therefore want to look at how you can apply this material to your wider life experiences and to adapt, combine and use it in ways that make sense for you in a more general way.

Michael Walton
1995

PART ONE:
CONCEPTS, CARE AND CONTEXT

Trying to work out what is going on, in and around you, is difficult unless you have some way of ordering your experiences and perceptions. The purpose of this part is to set out some initial frameworks that you can use. It will offer a means to build on as you work your way through the book and give you a way to order and put into context your experiences and observations.

Working with others is also a difficult and complicated business. It is not as straightforward or as easy as we are often led to believe. This is where we start. Chapter 1 introduces some initial ideas about the complexity of human interactions and the difficulties each of us experiences when working with others.

Chapter 2 provides a brief outline history of the NHS. Knowing even a little about the background history of your workplace can help you to understand some of the current issues and quirks! By looking at the history of the organization it can help you make more sense of what you are doing there.

The final chapter in this part looks at formal organizations. Most of us work in organizations of one sort or another. If you have a framework that you can use to understand your organization, it can be very helpful. You can apply these perspectives very easily to non-NHS settings and in so doing you will probably learn even more about the NHS at large, and your part of it in particular.

Chapter 1
The Dynamics of the Social World

Subjective understandings

When people come together interpersonal communications are initiated at several levels of awareness simultaneously. These range from openly expressed verbal communications, to messages communicated through intuition or body language, to those subliminal communications of which both the sender and the receiver are not consciously aware. These *dynamics* form the core of what it means to be a person in relation to someone else and, depending on the nature of these dynamic interactions, will determine what we say, feel and do.

Working with other people *is* complicated and this is often forgotten, or downplayed. Human communications are more than their expressed content suggests because they are the result of us having assessed and summed up the situation in front of us and decided (consciously and unconsciously) upon a course of action. Unexpressed and unconscious communications in particular exert an enormous influence on what goes on between people and on what decisions are taken and should therefore be considered more often than I believe is currently the case.

A heightened awareness of the unexpressed dimensions of our relationships and communications with others will remind you to look beyond what is said, or done. It will also help you to consider other dynamics that might hold the clue to establishing more effective relationships. It is similar to a patient asking for advice or guidance about a matter that you know they are familiar with but which they are using to mask another, possibly deeper, concern which will subsequently become more apparent as you work with them.

Over a period of time we each build up our own unique understanding of the social world around us based on what we have been told, what we see others doing and on our experiences. In this way we create our own individual 'world view' into which we then *fit* our subsequent experiences – and this is the same process for those around us – we all have our own subjective worlds, each different from the other.

The critical significance of this is that we will attribute different meanings – based on our views on matters – to occurrences we have shared with others. Most of the time these differences do not surface and we are able to work with others with relative ease and with mutual accommodation. Yet our different perceptions at times do lead to disagreements, misunderstandings and conflict. As far as each person is concerned though they are 'right' because their conclusions are based on their subjective view of what is going on. They will always see and make sense of things through their own 'eyes'. In health care settings, where anxiety levels are higher than normal, patients are very likely to feel under some psychological threat and can react defensively when they perceive their subjective view of the world being challenged. Unless you keep the points noted above in the forefront of your mind you too may respond defensively rather than seeking to understand and determine the cause of patient anxiety. You need to recognize that they will probably have a very different view about what is going on to yours.

If you can try to find out where the differences are – and where the problems seem to lie – you have more of a chance of resolving the differences together and of building mutual understanding. The key point is that while we share many of our perceptions with others the meanings we give to them can be very different. Now, if I'm your patient I will probably remain wary or suspicious of you unless you try to understand my view of what is going on. Easier said than done though. It takes time and effort and you have to hold in check your own issues, concerns and biases to do this well.

Being under tension and stress affects what we see, retain, and act upon. It also affects what we miss, discard, view as unimportant and choose to discount. The views and perceptions we hold about ourselves also influence our perceptions of external events and how we respond to situations. Tension with others is generated by many different factors some of which are noted in Fig. 1.1.

Before you read any further what additional sources of interpersonal stress and tension would you include from your experience using Fig. 1.1. as a prompt?

Now when you look at the features I have highlighted in Fig. 1.1 (together with those you have added) many of them relate to interpersonal *dynamics*. Such tensions and anxieties arise because people do not always see things the same way or agree on what needs to be done. We each reach our own conclusions about what we want, or do not want to happen. We then start behaving in ways which reflect the outcomes we want. These tensions and stresses arise because each one of us is following a similar process. Because it will not always be possible to meet each person's wishes, some will be disappointed and frustrated by not getting what they want. In addition, each of us has differing tolerances for handling personal disappointment and for coping with the uncertainty this creates. This in turn creates more tension and anxiety.

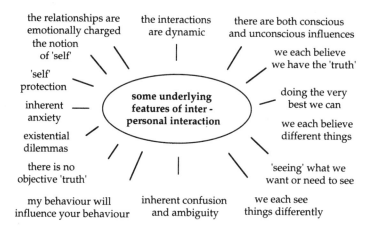

the relationships are emotionally charged

the notion of 'self'

'self' protection

inherent anxiety

existential dilemmas

there is no objective 'truth'

my behaviour will influence your behaviour

the interactions are dynamic

inherent confusion and ambiguity

there are both conscious and unconscious influences

we each believe we have the 'truth'

doing the very best we can

we each believe different things

'seeing' what we want or need to see

we each see things differently

some underlying features of inter-personal interaction

Fig. 1.1 Some sources of interpersonal tension.

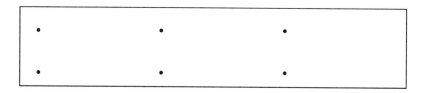

Fig. 1.2 Additional sources of interpersonal tension.

In clinical settings – where the whole context itself is anxiety provoking – these interpersonal worries, tensions and stresses are rapidly generated and displayed. It is little wonder that patients (and nurses too) get worried, seem to 'over-react' to little things and are terrified of asking the questions they want the answers to.

What can I hold on to?

To cope with such underlying pressures – and to look after yourself (and your patients) at the same time – takes strength, personal insight and energy. One way of doing this is to know who you are, what you stand for, and the values and beliefs that you hold dear. Clarifying what you believe in is not an easy thing to do, but you can make a start by noting down the beliefs, values and ways of working that seem to make sense to you. The items you make a note of need not all be to your liking, or philanthropic or 'worthy' ones; that doesn't make them any less important to know about or acknowledge. Being human is not about trying to be 'perfect' but about seeing yourself as you really are. This includes those aspects that both please and displease you.

You can amass quite a lot of information about a person, by listening to them, looking at them and also noticing how they present themselves. There are also many other less apparent layers of meaning that are not readily available for inspection. One way of thinking about this is to imagine youself as layers of an onion. You know that onions have many layers of 'skin'. In the same way there are many different layers of you with the core being tucked away right at the heart of the onion. It is from this core that subsequent growth, individual characteristics and the external shape are formed. The message here is that no one can know or understand a person solely through the information they externalise, they need to pay attention to what may be at the heart of that person if they want to appreciate and understand them more fully.

If I want to understand you, I have to move somehow beyond the outer shape and the protective layers that have been built up over the years towards the inner core; and I can only do this ethically if you wish it to happen and are willing to work with me. It is the same for ourselves; if we want to know a little more about why we do what we do we have to get through the protective layers we have put in place. The knowledge and understanding we reach can lead us to make changes here and there if we think it appropriate and, at the same time, reinforce other aspects of our beliefs and ways of being.

Figure 1.3 shows an onion skin model of self which shows several different 'levels' of self, ranging from what others 'see' me to be, to my most personal and private values and views on things which are right at the middle.

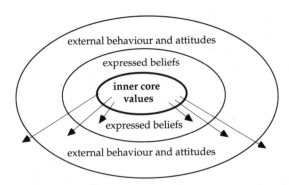

Fig. 1.3   An onion skin model of self.

So, at the core of you are your deeply held beliefs – most of which you may be unclear about but which guide, drive and influence (i) what you say you believe in; (ii) how you 'see' yourself; (iii) how you behave and (iv) the attitudes you express.

You may get a clue about some of your core values and beliefs if you take a moment to reflect during times when you are emotionally intense. For example, try to get behind *why* you sometimes feel overly threatened or challenged by someone else's point of view. You know from your own experiences how, at times, you can feel very challenged when asked to alter your view or position on a matter. In other cases a similar challenge seems to matter little to you. It is likely that in the first instance you felt one of your core values or views on life was under threat in some way, which then mobilized a defensive reaction from you. In the second instance perhaps the change required was less important to you. It did not threaten some aspects of you that you hold dear and thus needed no protective response.

Just as it is with you, so it is the same with other people. Sometimes you want them to change their behaviour and it is no problem at all – they just do it with no apparent difficulty or resistance at all. At other times it starts to feel as if a major war has erupted; you begin to wonder what it was you asked them to change because their response seemed out of proportion to the request or directive you made. It may be in some cases of extreme resistance or reaction that you touched an aspect of that person's self view that was important to them. If they were to change their position on that matter, they would experience a loss of some inner part of themselves – so, not surprisingly, they strongly resist.

My behaviour/your behaviour

One of the most significant determining factors in the shaping of relationships is your own individual *behaviour* because it conditions the consequent behaviour you receive from others. For example, in order for me to begin to relate in a meaningful way to you I need something on which to base my actions and decisions. That something is your behaviour as, at least initially, that is all I have to go on. I am defining behaviour here to cover all the ways you have chosen to present yourself to the outside world.

My interpretation of your behaviour thus influences how *I* then behave towards you and so the spiral of cause and effect continues with us each influencing each other. As I get to know you better I begin to realize that how you sometimes behave is not a very accurate reflection of who you are or what you want. But until we have built up some mutual understandings, and trust, I will respond to my interpretation of the behaviour you (or your patients, colleagues etc.) exhibit. That is the best I can do. In relation to the onion skin diagram (Fig. 1.3) I am responding to some of your outer skin behaviours because I don't yet know what lies beneath them – your beliefs – and I certainly have little idea of what is at the core of you.

Perhaps you can recall situations when you observed one of your colleagues being cooperative, helpful and pleasant with one person but then, strangely perhaps, offhand, less cooperative and less helpful with the next patient. In reflecting on this do you recall what may have led your colleague to treat these two people so differently? It may have been due to the different behaviour your colleague received from the people involved or as a consequence of his behaviour towards them.

Can you recall examples from your own experience where how you were treated (in the non-clinical sense) by patients caused you to behave differently towards them? I don't mean that the care that you delivered was inappropriate or mean, although of course it could have been, but where how you interacted with them was, somehow, markedly different (Fig. 1.4). What do you think were the factors that led you to behave differently towards them? Use the headings in Fig. 1.4 to record your reflections.

Patient/Colleague	The episode	My behaviour	Reasons why

Fig. 1.4   Some reflections on my behaviour.

It is very likely that it was something about how you both behaved towards each other that influenced the pattern of responses between you. Their behaviour, in effect, causing to some extent your behaviour. So it should not be unexpected that confronted with a patient who is being argumentative and uncomplimentary in some way you would want to respond in a defensive, terse way. Or else you would try to speed up the treatment so that you get away from them as soon as you can. In doing so however, you may miss the opportunity to find out why they are behaving in that way, and what you could consider doing differently in the future.

Equally it may strike you how much you prefer to attend to another patient's requests with great speed and that you listen very carefully to what they say. It is very probable that you are responding to the behaviour they are exhibiting towards you. You may not realize the extent to which you are doing this.

See if this makes sense next time you are working with colleagues or patients. Notice if your behaviour towards them seems to have any conditioning effect on how they behave towards you. How you come across to others influences their *perception* of you. In turn it influences their behaviour as a response to yours. As far as others are concerned all they see of you is your behaviour. This will lead them to a view that *you are your behaviour and your appearance*. They have little else to work from until they begin to know you better.

What is the 'truth' then?

This raises the question of what to believe about others and about oneself. Is there a single 'you' or are you made up of an infinite variety of selves? The question of the truth also arises; after all you may ask what am I to believe in? Often we operate as if there is always a definite 'truth' to situations, issues, meanings. We may consider that there will therefore be *right* decisions that need to be taken and *wrong* ones to be avoided. I am not talking here of clinical decisions about treatment but about interactions between people. This lack of certainty in human matters is often skated over because it is very reassuring to believe that you know the answer. It is also disconcerting to acknowledge that very few things within human relationships and well-being are cast in stone.

The trouble though, or the joy perhaps, is that there are many truths. It all depends on what you are looking for and the position from which you are observing and experiencing matters. One dramatic implication from this is that there can be no single interpretation of a situation experienced by several people. Each person brings with them their own uniquely formed view of things. While there may well be considerable overlapping of values, perspectives, and beliefs there will always be differences at some point between one person and another.

This is a vital understanding to take into account when working with patients, and colleagues. Each of us will invariably prefer to see things from our own perspective. In terms of your caring for others therefore do not assume that the patient (or anyone else) will see it your way or reach the same conclusions as you even though the data you are working from is the same. It is the sense each person makes of it, and the position they are operating from which are the unknown factors. To relate in an understanding and sensitive way requires you to take account of how someone else sees their situation (their truth if you like) as well as how you see it (your truth).

Figure 1.5 represents two people starting to work with each other – perhaps in order to reach a decision or make sense of some figures, etc.

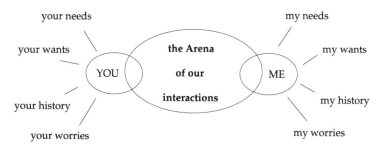

Fig. 1.5 Behind the face-to-face contact.

It indicates some of the background considerations that each party brings with them into that interaction. I have highlighted four background areas. Add others as they occur to you that will have an effect in shaping how they present themselves and what they will seek to secure from this interaction.

My own personal needs, wants, my history and my worries and anxieties will all come with me into this engagement. Even though we may be talking about a specific item on a formal agenda these aspects of me will also be there influencing what I do and how I react. It will be the same for you too.

Remember, when you are working with others – especially patients and clients – what they present and what you see before you is not necessarily the complete story. This means that you cannot rely solely on what is overtly presented to you. You should be prepared to consider more deeply the needs, wants, history and worries of your patients.

Think back to a recent meeting or discussion when you found that you were a little confused or perplexed by some of the reactions you received from your patients or colleagues. You could use the diagram as an initial step in clarifying what may have been going on and where the reactions, or difficulties you experienced could have been coming from.

To make a start note down what you know about each of the headings on Fig. 1.6 about (1) you, (2) them, (3) the setting and (4) the particular situation involved (these could be linked to your specific tasks). See if this throws any more light on what you experienced (or are currently experiencing). If you have added other dimensions please make notes about them too.

You can use this figure to speculate what sorts of needs, worries, etc.,

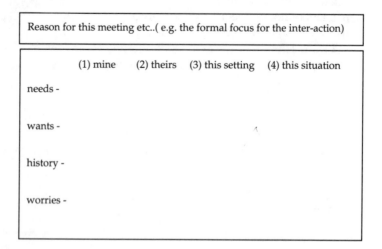

Fig. 1.6 Preparing for the interaction.

the other person may be bringing with them. This can then help you address them, or remind you to explain or ask about particular things you anticipate may be on their minds. These will vary from patient to patient, from setting to setting and from time to time. As you do this type of preparation, by making a note of your concerns and intentions, you will be more aware of your own issues and dilemmas.

You may begin to see, for example, that there is a clash of wants and needs between the two of you. Or perhaps the context (the ward or clinic) has a special meaning for either you or the patient which is affecting things. Perhaps the task you are to perform has an important symbolic meaning and importance to you, the patient, your colleague or all of you. You may therefore want to suggest an alternative setting to meet in or some other change which will facilitate a successful outcome of your work.

You can use your notes and reflections to try to clarify what was going on and the part you played in it. Getting into the habit of doing this will help you understand situations and help you to cope better, and anticipate problems, next time. Most importantly, it will be beneficial for enhancing the care you give to your patient and also to yourself.

Figure 1.6 highlights the likelihood that we can't expect everyone to see things exactly as we do. While they will have similar needs, motivations and wants as your own they will also see some things differently too. You just need to recognize this when working with others.

Levels of communication

As you look more deeply at interpersonal communications not only does it become clear that what we do (in our thinking and in our behaviour) rests in some way on previous experiences but that, in addition, we are not fully aware of everything about ourselves. There are, at least, three levels of communication that are activated when we are with other people. Acknowledging this can help you to anticipate problems. For example, there are:

(1) the communications that we hear and take part in with others openly,
(2) those communications and understandings known only to some of those around us and which are kept hidden from those 'not in the know' etc., and
(3) the unconscious patterns of communication about which neither we nor others have direct knowledge but which we sense indirectly.

An example of the last point would be where you find yourself doing something slightly out of character for you. You may say to yourself 'I wonder why I did that?'. Perhaps you are carried along with something you would not *normally* say or do etc. and you are puzzled and a little uneasy about why this happened. These could be examples of behaviour that arose because of unconscious motivations or needs that were activated.

Three main levels of communication then to keep in mind are shown in Fig. 1.7.

Level One: Manifest Behaviour & Processes

Level Two: Covert Behaviour & Processes

Level Three: Unconscious & Processes

Fig. 1.7 Levels of communication.

The three levels are active at the same time even though you might consciously be operating on the basis of level one predominantly, and then with level two for some of the time. These three levels can remind you to take a wider view when you are working with others. They can also remind you that there will be communications going on (level three) that affect what you are doing of which you (and others) have no conscious awareness.

Such phenomena affect nursing practice in several influential, but often unrecognized, ways. They influence how the nurse feels and the nature of the nurse–patient relationship. What then are the consequences for nursing practice if:

- people are guided by their private inner beliefs,
- we each 'see' and 'experience' things differently,
- there is no objective truth so far as 'feelings' are concerned,
- there are hidden and obscured levels of communication?

You may like to jot down your own thoughts about this but the main messages I take from these points are that:

- the nurse–patient interaction is not a straightforward, simple and rational one,
- that you and your patient will experience shared experiences differently,
- that you are likely to emphasize different aspects of those shared experiences,
- the nurse–patient relationship carries a high potential for interpersonal disharmony, misunderstanding and confusion,

- unless these factors are applied in your practice the likelihood of increased stress is heightened.

What adds to the complexity and ambiguity of the caring relationship is that while the nurse and the patient will experience matters differently, such differences may neither be verbalized or apparent. On the surface all may appear to be normal.

As a nurse, or as another care provider, this means you need to note not only what the patient says and does but also what they don't say. Do not assume that all is well purely on the basis of what they initially say to you. For yourself the implication is to acknowledge your responses and feelings more fully and later to discuss them with a colleague.

The dynamics of the relationships that you have with your patients and colleagues dramatically affect how you go about your work, your sense of well-being, and your self-confidence. In order to use your clinical skills to full effect you will need to pay attention to these aspects of your life.

The special role of the carer

The role of the nurse is quite special. I don't mean by this that it is precious in an exclusive way, but that the nurse–carer is in a very intimate and privileged relationship not only with the care–receiver but with other colleagues too. While there is nothing new in this statement, I believe it can often become lost in the routines and pressures of daily care.

You as the nurse matter a great deal to the patient. For the nurse it can be all too easy to – partly to protect oneself – categorize patients by their condition; generalize about relatives and stereotype the professional reactions of one's colleagues and, in so doing, blunt the edge of that essential quality of clinical nursing care *the qualitative relationship*. Closeness, intimacy, familiarity and their accompanying emotional intensity can lead to demands and pressures which are difficult for the nurse and her patient to handle.

The continuity of nursing care is quite different from the episodic care provided by other health care professionals. It often leads to a relationship between the nurse–carer and those being cared for that has immense psychological impact on both parties. The feelings aroused can go to the emotional extremes of intensely positive and intensely negative feelings. They can arise from the closeness and the mutual dependency and vulnerability of the relationship.

The intensity of these emotional attachments can spill over and influence the professional care of the patient. Both the patient and the nurse can be vulnerable to being cast by the other as either 'too good' or 'too bad'. As so much emotional intensity is generated and strong feelings and attachments are made, *how* these are acknowledged and handled are matters of considerable importance for the good health and care of patients and their carers.

The carer role offers immense psychological rewards. It also holds considerable potential for tension, confusion and transgressions of trust. It allows privileged access to the personal and private worlds of others and is also matched by a physical intimacy that pushes and pulls carer and patient close together. Yet at the same time it threatens to pull them apart unless such matters are regularly considered as part of the nurse's professional development.

Such intensely personal and emotive relationships result in a bonding (or a violent adverse reaction) which the nurse has to contend with daily and with several patients. This may be one of the reasons why the nursing role is such a personally rich and satisfying one and may also be why it is so stressful. When brought together, the combination of the physical, intellectual, emotional and technical demands that are made represent considerable strain and lead to high expectations of the nurse to meet all of these demands.

One way of easing the combined pressure this creates is to look at what is going on within the caring relationship and to clarify the expectations you hold for yourself and those which others may expect of you.

Great expectations

What do you believe patients expect of you as a nurse? Certainly the patient expects a professional diagnosis, some decisions to be made about the necessary treatment and then these decisions to be followed through in an appropriately professional, rigorous, safe and humane manner. The patient probably expects some prognosis too about the future for them and information from you about how their time as an in-patient will be spent. They will want information about their care in hospital and about the follow-up arrangements after discharge. They will probably be worried about post-operative care, the side-effects of drugs, possibly about coping with the loss of a part of their physical body, or of their state of mind. They will also be preoccupied about cure, mortality and their future prospects. They will want to know what the doctor meant, and what you think. Some may also want to keep in touch with you socially after discharge.

But each patient has expectations of another kind. They will have expectations about *you as a person*, not the you they see as the pro-fessional but about what you will do for them as another human being. They will draw on their past experiences, on folklore, on what people have said about your clinic, your ward, your speciality – maybe even about you in person. They will recall films about hospitals and GP practices, about documentaries on the NHS and on private medicine, and they will conjure up images from their imagination of what nurses are and what they do to people.

They will be nervous and worried and this will interfere with their view of what is going on. They are likely to read more meaning in what you say to them (which can be very different from the words you actually used). They are susceptible to misinterpret their situation and your motives and intentions.

These are important factors which have to be taken into account in your practice and they will colour the perceptions of the care expected by your patients and the care you provide. One way is to be aware just how susceptible they are to misperceiving their situation and for you to work accordingly. Remove ambiguities from what you say and check their understanding of what you have said. If you don't do this you leave the door open to confusion, complaints and avoidable distress – for you as well as the patient.

Another way is to be as clear as you can be about the expectations patients, relatives, and others are

- likely to be holding about you
- about the type of work you do and perhaps
- the profession as a whole.

If you can do this you create a basis from which to make more sense of what the patient is looking for, whether it is realistic or not.

If you are unable to build up a realistic mutual understanding, this can cause frustration and impede patient care and recovery. Being clearer about the expectations others have of you does not mean they will be realistic, valid, or possible to deliver. But at least if you know what they are expecting you can begin to reshape them to more appropriate and manageable ones (see Chapter 7 for a more detailed exploration of these matters).

Further reading

Honey, P. (1992) *Problem People*. Institute of Personnel Management, London.

Kagan, C., Evans, J. and Kay, B. (1986) *A Manual of Interpersonal Skills for Nurses*. Harper and Row, London.

McCrone, J. (1993) *The Myth of Irrationality*. Macmillan, London.

Sutherland, S. (1992) *Irrationality: the enemy within*. Constable, London.

Walton, M.J. (1984) *Management and Managing*. Harper and Row, London.

Watzlawick, P. (1976) *How real is real?* Vintage Books, New York.

Chapter 2
Overview of the NHS

Taking the patient's history is an important step and much can be gleaned from talking to the patient. A patient's background can alert you to look for particular symptoms and allow you to be prepared for expectations they may have. It will prepare you for reactions you think likely because of past treatments, and set you thinking about future needs because of health patterns in the patient's family. However, too much emphasis on what has gone before can overburden, confuse and blind you to the current needs of the patient, which may have been pushed aside.

The same situation applies to organizations. A knowledge and an understanding of their past can help you to understand what is going on today. They have a history that needs to be taken into account, just as a patient has. A great deal of the issues, conflicts, dilemmas and rivalries you see today may have their origins in the events of many years ago. Knowing why particular patterns of organizational behaviour are occurring is no guarantee that such behaviour will be easily altered. In fact, some of the most intriguing situations are those where there is general consent about the need for change but where – for some reason or other – nothing does change! This is a theme explored in Part Four.

However, an understanding of the background history can lead you to propose actions that take into account some of the underlying deeper ailments within the organization and not solely to focus on superficial cosmetic issues. By knowing the history we have some basis for looking anew at how situations have arisen and we can then adopt sensible ways of changing things for the future.

With an organization like the NHS it is possible to trace the changes in its overall structure up to the present time. Doing this will show how it was set up and some of the major policy initiatives that have underpinned the structural changes.

Remember that the NHS is one of the most complicated, and largest, organizations in the world. It is generally well regarded for the work it does, but it has its problems. There are considerable variations, at hospital and clinic level, in service provision and resource allocations. One of the confusing things I find about the service is this variation. One moment you can be in a leading edge, well resourced department and the next in a location where more resources are sorely needed and yet both are part of the same NHS.

Our NHS is rarely out of public attention and it remains a service which attracts intense political debate and attention. The degree of public attention, and political intrusion, it receives generates additional anxiety and stress which it can well do without.

Inception of the NHS

The NHS came into being on 5 July 1948 following the passing of the National Health Service Act of 1946. In England and Wales the legislation required the Minister of Health

> To promote the establishment of a comprehensive health service designed to secure improvement in the physical and mental health of the people and the prevention, diagnosis and treatment of illness, and for that purpose to provide or secure the effective provision of resources.

Similar provisions were made for Scotland and Northern Ireland.

While the stated purpose of the NHS was to provide a comprehensive health service for all, improving the physical and mental health of the nation and the prevention, diagnosis and treatment of illness was an enormous undertaking. The NHS was originally set up as three service sectors: hospital services, primary care and local authority services. There was little coordination between these sectors and it was the high profile hospital sector that received most attention and had the largest budget.

The original structure is shown in Fig. 2.1 and it persisted in this pattern for some 26 years. There was a large coordination, and resource allocation, gap between the hospitals sector and the primary care and local authority services. Moves towards a more integrated and streamlined NHS structure were finally taken with the 1974 reorganization when an attempt was made to integrate hospital and community-based services more fully. Even though those in general practice remained outside the new health authorities, provision was made for them in the legislation to be members of the new management teams.

The reorganization created new area health authorities, each with health districts under them, with one (or more) district general hospitals as the centrepiece for the integration of local health services. Each health district was managed by a district management team, which, for the first time, included two elected medical representatives, a hospital consultant and a GP, in addition to a formally appointed district medical officer. The former local authority medical officer of health services were disbanded and integrated within the new health authorities. In the

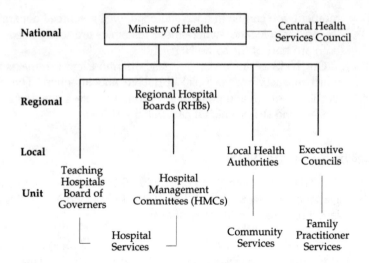

Fig. 2.1   The NHS 1948–1974 (a simplified diagram).

primary care sector however, the GPs remained separately funded and were serviced under a local family practitioner committee which served the same patient catchment area as the health authority. Figure 2.2 shows how the new structure looked.

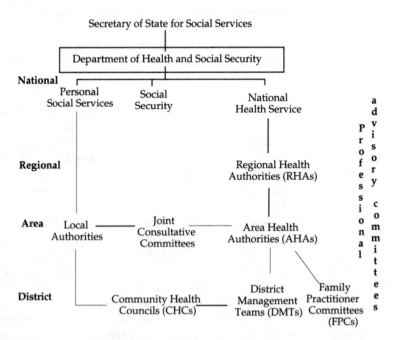

Fig. 2.2   The reorganized NHS in 1974 (simplified).

This reorganization represented a determined move towards a more integrated health service but it was not completely achieved and the gap between hospital, local authority and GP services has remained wide. It was at this time that a new body – the community health council (CHCs) – came into being. Its aim was to give patients a stronger local voice and provide a vehicle through which advocates for the relatively neglected care services (e.g. the elderly or the mentally ill) could be more formally, and more forcefully, heard.

The new area health authorities (AHAs) reported into 14 regional health authorities (RHAs) which in turn reported into the Department of Health and Social Security (DHSS). In the event, the administrative arrangements of this structure – which also set up a whole series of planning committees – proved to be too elaborate as did the *consensus management* system of decision making. The idea is sound but it is not valid if applied to every situation: sometimes one person must collect views and decide. In a complex organization like a hospital, consensus management universally applied is not quick or effective enough where there are many vested interests to satisfy. Increasing financial pressures also led to a dramatic change in how central funds were to be allocated. Up until 1976, when cash limits on public expenditure were introduced, resources had been allocated in proportion to previous expenditure allowing for a measure of (sometimes creeping and unmanaged) expansion. From 1976 an attempt was made to level out geographical disparities and imbalances in funding between different care groups. An attempt was also made to move more resources to the specialities seen as deprived .

In 1982 the area health authorities were replaced by 200 district health authorities (DHAs) which were given more autonomy in planning freedom for their patient catchment area. However, the annual performance review system was also introduced. By emphasizing targets and outputs that were centrally determined, it significantly constrained the relative autonomy that the 1982 change to DHAs had sought to achieve.

The Griffiths Report

Roy Griffiths was invited to give advice on the effective use and management of manpower and related resources in the service and led a team looking at these matters. The recommendations of the Griffiths Report (1983) were, in essence, to propose the introduction of a general management structure and philosophy throughout the NHS. An NHS management board was proposed and management was to be judged on its performance. The NHS would be looked at, and run, far more as a business concern than ever before.

The team saw the need, at all levels of the NHS, for a more integrated focus. This brought together all the activities involved in a more business-like way and directed the focus towards achieving defined targets and goals. What they saw was a lack of a general management process. The solution was to introduce this philosophy of a more business-like approach. General managers (regardless of their discipline) were introduced at regional, district and unit level. They were responsible for the effective leadership and management of their organizations and the introduction of a general management process throughout the service.

Consensus decision making, the fudging of difficult funding and resource issues, 'doing things the way we have always done' etc., would go. Competitive tendering was also introduced to test the cost efficiency and effectiveness of in-house services, such as catering, laundry and cleaning. The automatic dependence by hospitals on these internal 'hotel' services was to be market tested.

These changes were a watershed in the management of the NHS. They pulled it away from a legacy of consensus decision making (based on mutual collaboration and accommodation of differences) to the introduction – some would say imposition – of a general manager as the autonomous decision maker when all other options failed. This philosophy and approach was 'cascaded' throughout the organization and opened up prospects of a career to the very top management roles irrespective of one's professional discipline. What mattered was the ability to manage a multi-professional team in a professionalized working environment to agreed targets within agreed resources. Also a preparedness to be judged on your results at the end of your limited (usually three year) contract.

The internal market: purchasers and providers

The late 1980s saw a radical review of the NHS and its workings. It was decided to introduce into the NHS a form of market competition that was intended to stimulate the efficiency and effectiveness of health care services at their point of delivery. Over a period of time it would raise the standards of the service nationwide. The method selected to do this was to separate out those who were responsible for ensuring that the health needs of their population were properly provided for – *the purchasers* – from those who were commissioned to provide and deliver the care services to patients and clients – *the providers*.

Purchasing decisions would be made by the district health authorities or GPs who had been devolved funds and who would be allowed to manage their own budgets (GP fundholders). The providers – the hospitals, clinics and community-based services – would contract with purchasers to provide defined levels of service in exchange for a formal contract of service. A key dynamic of the new *internal market* system was that purchasers (DHAs and GPFHs) could choose where to put their business depending on the quality and the range of care services offered by interested providers.

After an initial period of settling down, purchasers would shop around to get the best services for their patient population with the money they had available. Providers, on the other hand, would have an incentive to provide the most effective and efficient services they could in order to secure their base funding with their historical purchaser. Then they would also contract to provide care services for purchasers they had not previously served. It was hoped that this element of (internal) market competition would ultimately bring benefits to all parts of the NHS system.

An increasing emphasis was placed on cost-effectiveness and cost improvements in all areas of NHS practice and organization. More emphasis was directed onto the management of clinical budgets and doctors were highlighted as being an integral and critical part of the management process. Clinical directorates were set up to integrate the work plans, expenditures and outputs of medical departments and to take collective medical responsibility for managing their affairs to meet agreed targets within the monies allocated. GPs too were given indicative drug targets and allowed more freedom to undertake – where viable and appropriate – cost-effective treatments in the surgery (e.g. day surgery). Hitherto this had been done in hospitals.

At the same time hospital and community services were given the opportunity to become independent in their own right and to opt for autonomous Trust status, subject to local consultation and the approval of the Secretary of State. This independence would allow more self-determination and free them from RHA direction and control although remaining obligated to national initiates such as *The Patients' Charter*, *Health of the Nation*, *Care in the Community* etc.

As providers, Trusts can choose to compete for business with other Trusts and directly managed units (DMUs) as a feature of the workings of the internal market. In spite of their separation from direct accountability to region, regional health authorities have kept an overview on the workings of the Trusts within their region and have exercised a discrete influence on Trust interactions and competitive intentions. It remains to be seen how this overview will be provided after regions have been disbanded – the next stage of the NHS reforms.

An outline of the current NHS structure is shown in Fig. 2.3.

The new management arrangements

Parliament's objective is to streamline the structure still further, and to maximize the proportion of the budget allocated to providing direct patient care. Significant changes to the existing (1995) arrangements

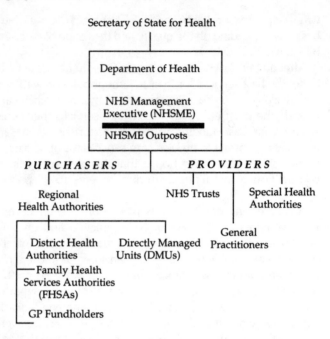

Fig. 2.3   Structure of the NHS in 1994.

have been announced although these will not be fully implemented until 1996 as they require Parliamentary approval.

The main changes are:

- the abolition of regional health authorities,
- their replacement by eight regional offices of the NHS Executive (no longer called the NHSME),
- the creation of larger health 'commissioning agencies' integrating the work of the former DHAs and FHSAs.

The proposed structure is shown in Fig. 2.4.

The NHS has been in a state of continuing evolutionary change for most of its history. Yet the most far reaching set of changes appear to have occurred in the last decade following the Griffiths Report and the introduction of a general management philosophy. The pressure for change has not always arisen from within the DHSS or the DoH. But it has arisen from a wider governmental responsibility to make the best use of the massive funding that goes into the NHS and in response to the external pressures on government funds (thus increasing pressure on the NHS budget).

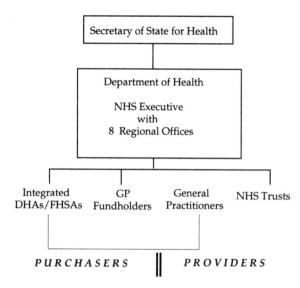

Fig. 2.4 The new structure of the NHS (with effect from 1996).

Management traditions within nursing

As with the overall structure of the NHS, the organization of nursing management has also had its fair share of changes over the years. Traditionally, the nursing organization centred around the matron. She was the principal nursing figure in all hospitals and for many, irrespective of their professional role, she was *the* key figure in any hospital. The trouble was that while this was *the* nursing title to have, the jobs varied greatly. Thus, something had to be done to achieve more definition of the seniority of the person called 'matron' .

For example, you would have a small cottage hospital with a matron, yet the same title could be used by a senior nurse manager in a major teaching hospital. This caused confusion within the profession and with non-nursing colleagues because it was often difficult to compare seniority and responsibility. Most of all the confusion was with patients and the public at large who had no way of easily differentiating between the various matron titles. Often all they wanted was to see the *matron*.

The Salmon Report (1966) was set up to enquire into 'the senior nursing staff structure in the hospital service (ward sister and above), the administrative functions of the respective grades and the methods of preparing staff to occupy them'. It was from 'Salmon' that the nursing officer structure originated (with grades from nursing officer to chief nursing officer being introduced), and nursing, teaching and midwifery *divisions* became the designated core specialisms in the new nursing organization.

The classification of the Salmon gradings is shown in Fig. 2.5. The report offered primarily an administrative and structurally oriented change. It also emphasized an increasing focus on the managerial and administrative responsibilities of senior nurses. By clustering clinical services into speciality areas or units – each of which could then have a nursing officer in charge – the changes offered scope for the ambitious clinically experienced nurse. While wanting more responsibility, nurses could also remain close to the patient. The changed structure offered a way to give more clinical responsibility without that nurse having to be promoted up into nursing administration which, up till now, had been the primary promotion route available.

Level	Number & title of grade	Local titles of posts
Top Management	10 Chief Nursing Officer(CNO)	Chief Nursing Officer, Principal
	9 Principal Nursing Officer (PNO)	Matron, Principal Tutor
Middle Management	8 Senior Nursing Officer (SNO)	Senior Matron, Senior Tutor, Senior Midwife Teacher
	7 Nursing Officer (NO)	Matron, Tutor, Midwife Teacher
First Line Management	6 Charge Nurse (CN)	Ward Sister, Section Sister, Midwifery Sister, Charge Nurse
	5 Staff Nurse (SN)	Staff Nurse, Staff Midwife

Fig. 2.5   The Salmon nursing structure.

The current senior nurse structure

With the advent of Trusts and the flexibility to determine pay structures locally there is no longer a nationwide pay structure to be formally followed. There are also no mandatory organization structures to adhere to with the exception of ensuring the provision of professional nursing advice to the Trust board. This can be done in a variety of ways. The most common way is by the appointment of directors of nursing (or clinical) services where the appointee is a trained and suitably experienced nurse.

An outline of the levels is shown in Fig. 2.6.

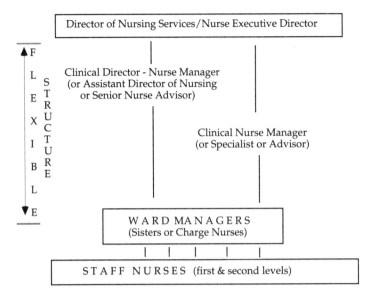

Fig. 2.6 Outline framework for nursing posts.

There is now considerable flexibity in the structure that can be put in place to organize and manage nursing services. In fact, the only fixed points are at the top level – where the Trust board must have professional nursing advice – and up to first level management with ward managers.

How the nursing structure is set up, between these two points, is for the Trust to decide and will reflect the local situation and the mix of services to be provided. As Trusts are using different job titles for similar levels of seniority, each organization structure will also need to be looked at separately, before any comparisons can be made, to define local usage and meaning.

Future changes

It has to be expected that the structure will continue to alter as time goes on. However, it may be that the most significant shifts are either already in place (i.e. the purchaser-provider split) or already signalled (e.g. the changes to regions and the moves towards fewer, larger commissioning authorities).

It is already possible for nurses to become general managers and reach very senior jobs in both Trusts and with purchasers. We have yet to feel the full effect of Project 2000 and the impact of pilot developments such as nurse practitioners and nurse prescribers. Each of these are major developments from the traditional positioning of the nurse within the NHS family.

I would expect that the pressure on outputs will continue. There will also be continuing efforts for the clinicians to accept even closer responsibility for the day-to-day management of their clinical resources and the development of clinical directorates.

References

NHS Management Inquiry (1983) The Griffiths Report, DHSS, London.
The Salmon Report on Senior Nursing Staff Structure (1966), HMSO, London.

Further reading

Ham, C. (1991) *The New National Health Service*, Radcliffe Medical Press Ltd, Oxford.
IHSM (1994) *The Health Services Year Book*, Institute of Health Services Management, London.
NAHAT Yearbook (1995) National Association of Health Authorities and Trusts.
Stewart, R. (1989) *Leading in the NHS*, Macmillan, London.
Teasdale, K. (1992) *Managing the Changes in Health Care* Wolfe Publishing Company, London.

Chapter 3
Organizations in Action

This chapter is about being in organizations, and my emphasis is on formal organizations. The chapter is written with the NHS in mind but you can very easily apply the material more generally to other settings if you wish to do so.

Most of us work in organizations but unfortunately working effectively and efficiently within them is not easy. Sadly, many people get damaged by their experiences and, from my experience, relatively few seem to really give of their best for much of their time at work. For some this can be because of a mismatch between the individual and the type of work they have elected to do. For others it can be the organization itself which seems to make it difficult to work productively and constructively.

Both of these scenarios are disturbing and dysfunctional for both the individual and their organization. There will invariably be difficulties in the individual organization interface and trying to work out why problems and difficulties are being experienced is a sound first step before deciding what needs to be done. It is intensely frustrating to feel that the organization is stopping you from doing your job. Or unreasonably, you may feel, that it is blocking your good ideas for changes that are obviously required, so that you cannot understand why no action has been taken.

If this is your experience look at how you are trying to get your ideas across to others, and understand why they seem to matter so much to you. Also try to diagnose how your part of the organization operates. This information will help you:

- decide if that is sufficient compatibility with your ways of working and values etc. for you to want to stay,
- identify the areas for possible change,
- assess the internal willingness and openness to change
- be more aware of what is important to you and, perhaps, why.

Many of us could do well to develop still further our understanding of organizational life and of how to remain effective in such work settings. While the future may offer more scope for independent self-employed practitioner status, you are still likely to be part of a small group and you

27

will still have to deal with other more formalized organisations. It is thus worthwhile understanding more fully how organizations are set up and how they work. Unless you decide to opt out in some way you will unavoidably have to think more about how organizations function, and how you can function well within them. This chapter offers some ideas about the nature of organizations and how make a start in assessing them.

Thinking about your organization

The nature, style and the tone of the organizations we work in profoundly affect our well-being and the quality of the work we do. It therefore surprises me that more attention is not given to thinking about how organizations are set up and what actually happens in practice.

By an organization I mean a group of suitably experienced and qualified people who work together in an ordered way. They work together for defined purposes and to achieve specified outcomes which require their combined efforts (e.g. to provide health care to a patient). It is not a random collection of people who suddenly turn up, but a very focused and carefully defined group of selected individuals.

The organization can be whatever size you decide to focus on; a clinical department, the ward, the Trust, the CMHT, the patients' records department or a health clinic. This chapter is about what it can mean to work within one of these formally constituted organizations. Wherever you are based you will be influenced in what you do, and how you do it, by the ethos and 'feel' of the health care organization you are a part of. You cannot escape the impact of organizational life.

This chapter will remind you to look at how your organization operates in practice. Often what is actually done is very different from what those at the top say will be done. Health care organizations at all levels differ a great deal and their particular nature and style will have a big effect on how you do your work, how you feel about it and whether you want to stay or move on. We also take a look at the notion of an organization having its own culture.

What is it like where you are?

To begin with, I would like you to start thinking about any organization that you are, or were until recently, a part of. You can then relate the material we cover to that organization and test out what I am saying against your own experience.

Decide on the organization you wish to focus on for this exercise. Choose one you know and have been in for at least a month or more because you need some history to draw on.

Step 1 – what's it like?

I want you to build up a picture – make an assessment – of your current situation. What comes into your mind when you begin to think about it. Make a note of your thoughts. Figure 3.1 contains a set of questions you can ask yourself as you build up the description.

---

1 Immediate Thoughts & Impressions that arise

2 What I like about it

3 What I dislike

4 What seems to matter here

5 What is not attended to or pushed aside

Fig. 3.1 Thinking about my organization.

Label these as your 'initial thoughts'. As this chapter progresses there will be additional thoughts and observations that you will want to record. You may want to be clear about your initial feelings and impressions to see if and how they change.

Step 2 – any underlying themes?

Now look at what you have recorded. Are there any underlying themes or patterns that you can identify from what you have written. Are there any hidden messages about your organization and how it functions? Are there any issues you know that are really important that you seem somehow to have missed or somehow just omitted from your notes? Why might that be? It could be that the most obvious things are easily forgotten, or overlooked. It could also be that it is easier at times to pretend that particular issues or concerns don't exist and are therefore best forgotten (particularly if others adopt the same strategy). Add any further thoughts to your notes.

Step 3 – any taboos and myths?

In thinking about where you work are there any topics or aspects of how the organization functions that people never seem to talk about? Have you been told not to ask about particular matters, or have you noticed that when certain things come up your colleagues go quiet etc? This could be because there are some areas of business that are taboo and by identifying these you can get invaluable information about the workings of your organization. Conversely are there any stories or is there mythology that is ritually handed down to newcomers – what are the organizational myths where you work?

Step 4 – what gets rewarded?

Are there particular behaviours that seem to be looked for, and are then rewarded. Conversely, are there ways of working or of 'being' that seem not to be encouraged, valued or wanted? If so what are they? Here again what you can pick up are the subtle shaping and conformity pressures that will reflect the nature and character of the organization in a way that an organization chart or a mission statement fails to do.

It can be very difficult to find out just who to believe, or what is actually going on in an organization. It is the same in politics where a lot of rhetoric is expressed. Where people pout and posture in ways intended to make people listen and believe them but where what you see is not always what you will actually receive. One way to find out is to become your own detective and to watch what the organization actually does rather than what it says it will do, and to use the above steps (1–4) to collect information that is often missed.

In one organization I know, developing the competence of professionals as managers was identified as *the* key priority. After a lot of talk and high-level meetings the appraisal procedure was altered to include a section on management skills and competencies. Seminars were held to demonstrate how much value was given to this important facet of a manager's job and it was stated that this would be one of the principal sections for consideration at the performance review meeting. It was largely all talk however. A manager's promotion and their financial and professional rewards continued to be based on their technical and professional skills, irrespective of how they managed their staff. Effective people management remained of little value in spite of all the forms and all the talking! Not surprisingly nothing changed and the poor use of highly skilled professionals continued unabated.

During the course of your work you can learn a great deal from just watching and noting what is actually rewarded and valued rather than relying on the expressed rhetoric. The latter is often intended to satisfy the internal politics and the outside observers of the organization. Don't forget to notice those behaviours, ways of doing things, rituals and procedures, forms of address etc. – that seem obvious to you. Others may not see them at all, or see them in a very different light.

By being detailed in this way you develop your ability to assess new situations and settings quickly. This gives you a more soundly based perspective.

Such observational and diagnostic skills will also help you to develop a clearer view of what to look for in your work settings and also what you don't want. If you don't develop these skills, you may find yourself inadvertently committed to working in settings where you are at odds with the organizational tone. You may experience stress that you could have avoided and come to wish you weren't there in the first place.

These four simple questions can elicit much information:

(1)   What's it like where you work?
(2)   What are the underlying themes?
(3)   What are the taboos and myths
(4)   What gets rewarded ?

You can respond to them as briefly or as fully as you want. They give you an uncomplicated initial framework for exploring your organization.

Take note of what is going on around you organizationally because there is a lot to see and few people take the time to look. The information you put together from these four questions, and any others you might want to use, can also help you to think more fully about your future career and what you want from your work.

What is likely to emerge from your notes is that formal organizations are not all they appear to be. They can work in unexpected ways which can be very confusing to their members (and to outsiders too).

It is highly likely that some of the working methods you currently follow are influenced more by what is locally acceptable (based in part on the history of that organization – see also Chapter 2) than the actual demands of the work to be done. You may have even identified, through the questions above, some cases where the most helpful behaviour is actually expressly outlawed or frowned upon. If this is the case, then one question is 'How can this be?' . . . or perhaps . . .'Are we unusual in this as an organization?' In the pages that follow you will be able to answer these questions for yourself.

What you have just completed is a partial diagnosis of your organization based on your observations and your direct experience of it. By looking once again at your everyday experiences you can begin to build up an assessment of what your organization is like, what it says and what it actually does and how it 'feels' to be there. Like all diagnoses it should remain a tentative hypothesis but you now have something to work from as you continue in your work and to keep an eye on as you observe what is going on around you.

Keep this initial diagnosis of your own organization in mind as you go through the rest of the chapter so that you can relate the material covered to it.

The notion of organizations

If you look at books on organizations the following characteristics appear to underpin most of what is written:

Organizations are:

- *Task focused:* they have been formed for a purpose and are there to get those things accomplished.
- *Logical-rational based:* generally they set about their work in an ordered, logical-rational way with procedures, processes and protocols intended to ensure that the desired tasks are completed appropriately
- *Exchange based:* there is some exchange made between the people involved in the work of the organization. It usually involves a mixture of financial, non-financial and psychological benefits in return for the person's time, effort, skills and commitment
- *Quantitative more than qualitative:* generally what matters are the tangible achievements rather than the quality of the working relationships to get the tasks done.
- *Identity, ethos and culture:* that organizations develop their own unique culture, style and tone that affects all who work within that setting. In effect organizations take on an identity and a character of their own

The emphasis is generally on tasks and order. The emotional dimensions are pushed to one side as if they do not need to be taken into account in the workings of the organization. This is surprising since organizations are primarily groups of people coming together to do different, but related tasks and who will bring with them their emotions and feelings as well as their specialist skills and knowledge.

It is also noticeable how, over a period of time, organizations seem to develop an identity of their own. Those within it often attach themselves to it with great commitment. This strong emotional attachment can then lead those inside an organization to defend it against any hint of criticism and threat even when such criticism may be justified. Sometimes organizations seem to take on a life of their own. They lose sight of their original aims, objectives and ethics to the extent that preserving the integrity (status, name, honour etc.) of the organization becomes more important than anything else.

I expect that you have noticed some of these features of organizational life already from your experience of the NHS or elsewhere. Such phenomena confirm to me just how complicated organizations are and how easy it is for them, and us inside them, to get mixed up and confused in what we do. Yet relatively little emphasis is given to these emotional, dynamic and interactional aspects of organizations. But more of this later.

Three organization models to use

To really look at your organization, you need to have a conceptual framework that you can use to think about the core functions which need to be undertaken. I have selected three ways of looking at organizations which illustrate the dynamics and relationships that exist within them. You can decide which makes most sense to you. I would like you to use one or more, in looking more closely at your organization to see how it functions.

At the heart of an organization should be the reason why it was put together in the first place; for the *work* it is there to do. Problems usually arise when this focus gets lost or when what began as ways of helping the work get done become more important than the work itself! If in confusion about issues, always see how what is being proposed relates, or not, to the stated core purpose of that organization. This gives you a starting point from which to assess the underlying problems and issues and how severe a state (how ill perhaps) that organization may be in.

Approach 1: Galbraith's 'fit' model (Galbraith, 1977)

This model emphasizes the interrelationships between five key areas of organizational functioning.

(1) To start with there is the *work* to be done and that should be the starting point for everything. We may decide we want a new clinic, or a hospital, or a community health centre – but what exactly do we want it to do?
(2) Once we have an answer and some clarity about the purpose we can then move on to consider what type of *structure* will be needed so that the results we are after can be achieved.
(3) With clarity about the structure we then have to decide what *people* will be needed to make it function.
(4) Then we must decide how we will pay and *reward* them.
(5) In order to know how we are doing, what adjustments to make, and what problems are arising etc. we have to then set up the *information* and *decision-making* arrangements that give us the information we require to make the organization operate effectively and efficiently.

The model is usually depicted as shown in Fig. 3.2. In this figure each component is shown as connected to all of the others because if any one is altered on its own the rest will go out of balance. The overall performance and effectiveness of the organization will thus be adversely affected. For example, suppose we are having problems staffing nights on a couple of wards and I make an executive decision

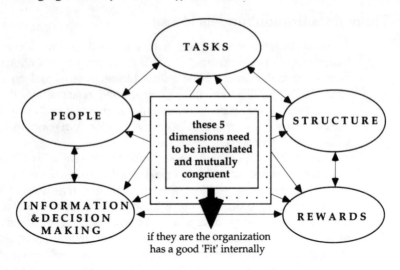

Fig. 3.2 Galbraith's 'fit' model.

to pay extra to make that duty more attractive and thus resolve my staffing problem. I may be able to do that through altering the *rewards* but it is likely that I will also create some internal friction with other staff (the *people*). They will also want an equal opportunity to get enhancements and those on nights elsewhere will want equity too. A further complication may be that when my decision is known – through the flow of management information – this could generate further problems if in reaching my decision I had somehow exceeded my authority.

An effective and well-performing organization is like a series of springs that are linked together to support something and which are in balance together. When a change is made to one part of that system – such as when the tension on one of the springs is altered – the others move in order to compensate. Even though they were not directly changed, they still have to move to find a new overall balance point to keep the organization (of springs) in balance.

So, you may decide to change the structure in an organization, or change the people. However, the rest of the system will also need to be readjusted and realigned if you want it to work effectively, efficiently and in balance. Often this is not done and the organization is thrown out of balance.

The important message is that the five dimensions (in Fig. 3.2) need to be in balance and mutually supporting each other, they need to 'fit' together. If you change any one of them on their own watch for 'knock-on' problems elsewhere.

Approach 2: The 7-S McKinsey model

This model came out of a very popular book called *In Search of Excellence* (Peters & Waterman, 1982) and identified seven key variables that needed to be considered in an interdependent way in any organization. It became known as the McKinsey 7-S framework and is shown in Fig. 3.3.

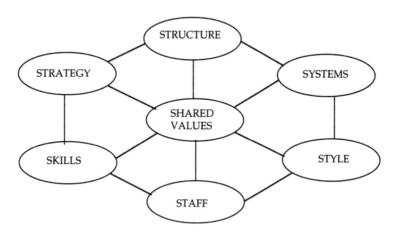

Fig. 3.3   The McKinsey 7-S model

The most interesting feature of this framework is that it highlights the importance of the softer aspects of management such as shared values and style which have not traditionally been focused upon. As with Galbraith's model, all these dimensions need attention and the message again is that you can't change one without affecting the others in some way.

The framework is a reminder to keep in mind the organization as a whole when you consider making changes (see also Part Four) and at the heart of it all are the shared values (cultural aspects) that will help to bind the organization together.

Approach 3: Weisbord's six-box model

This last framework comes from Marvin Weisbord (1978) (a well-known organization consultant); he has found it helpful in looking at an organization. He calls it the 'six-box model' and each of the boxes is used to look at a particular aspect of the formal and informal organization (see Fig. 3.4).

You can use the model to review things and to see if there are likely to be blockages or problems, either in the boxes themselves, or in their

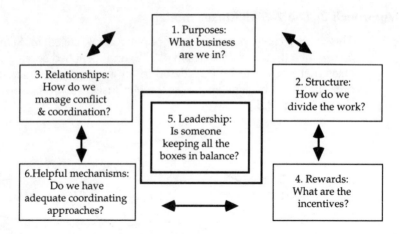

Fig. 3.4   Weisbord's six-box-model.

links to one another. Again, no one aspect of the organization is looked at in isolation, everything is seen as integrated.

As a straightforward, jargon-free approach it works well. It can be used to build up an overall picture onto which you could then add other dimensions, either from this chapter or from the material in Part Three, to make it more comprehensive.

What goes on in organizations: some perspectives to consider

Formal aspects of your organization

If you ask people to describe an organization they will probably begin to describe some of the formal aspects such as its structure, job titles, reporting relationships and grades and levels of staff. These are all important facets as they often provide the infrastructure for work to be undertaken. These will be the things that most people will concentrate upon and most of the reported difficulties and disputes are described in terms of these dimensions – grading and pay disputes, role confusion and reporting disputes, competition for formal power, and who is more senior to whom.

In continuing the diagnosis of your organization look at Fig. 3.5. What you may find is some confusion between how you are told some of these matters should be undertaken and resolved and what you have seen happen in practice. You may be noting how the formal organization structure – the way people say the organization should function – does not totally mirror the way the place actually operates. What you are now picking up are aspects of the *informal* organization at work.

(a) re: levels of formal authority:	for each of these (a) - (d) look
	to see how these aspects of
(b) re: roles and responsibilities	your organisation are set up;
	how formally the decisions
(c) re: hierarchy of decision-making	are meant to be made; and what
	the formal arrangements for
(d)re: patterns of payment & reward	managing the organisation are

Fig. 3.5   Questions to consider.

Less formalized aspects of your organization

It is very convenient to have a neat organization structure which is backed up by carefully worded practices that purport to codify and show how the place works. However organizations develop their own informal ways of working, some of which are in line with the formal organization and some of which run counter to it.

We develop our own informal patterns of influence, power and authority. We find out very quickly who to go to for reliable professional guidance and support, and we find out who are the informal leaders in the organization. We often go to them to get things done, or at least keep them informed about what is going on.

These are the additional ways in which the organization functions as opposed to only following the formally presented ways in which things are supposed to happen. If you now move your attention to the informal aspects of your organization there are three more questions to consider in Fig. 3.6.

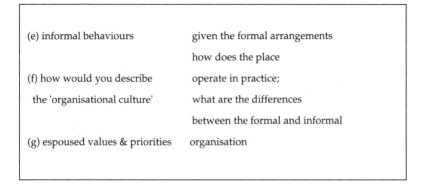

Fig. 3.6   More questions to consider.

Much of what really matters within the organization is bound up with the culture it has evolved. For example, whereas one hospital (clinic, clinical placement, ward etc.) can be a joy to work in, another – seemingly the same to all intents and purposes – can be hell. Much of what makes the difference can be attributed to the culture of that organizational setting, which can be driven by top and senior management, and influenced by external pressures.

Organizational culture

It is strange, but sometimes you can walk into a hospital or onto a ward and you immediately sense something about the place. You start to make assumptions about what it would be like to work there. Noticing the way the people behave, the types of interactions that go on between them and the way they relate to you gives you more information to add to your initial perceptions. After a brief period of time you can build up a rich picture of that place.

What you have been picking up are pieces of information about the culture of that organization – from the positioning (or absence even) of notices and directional signs, to the feel, smell and state of the place. Irrespective of all the formal information you may have received beforehand, being there is the key. It is amazing how varied, and numerous, these cultural messages are when you start to look for them and they can tell you so much.

The word 'culture' is conventionally used to describe the customs and behaviours of different lands and peoples. It may seem unusual to use the same concept to describe an organization such as a hospital or a health clinic. Yet it is an apt way of capturing the essence of an organization that is, after all, a separate community in its own right.

Some of the ways organizational culture has been described are as follows:

- 'how things are done around here' (Ouchi & Johnson, 1978),
- the values and expectations which organization members come to share (Van Maanen & Schein, 1988),
- the ways of thinking, speaking and acting that characterize certain groups (Braten, 1983),
- the 'taken for granted' and shared meanings that people assign to their social surroundings (Wilkins, 1983),
- the collection of traditions, values, policies, beliefs and attitudes that constitute a pervasive context for everything we do and think in an organization (McLean & Marshall, 1983).

One of the most intriguing comments about this comes from Edward Hall (1959) who observes how

... culture hides much more than it reveals and, strangely enough, what it hides, it hides most effectively from its own participants. Years of study have convinced me that the real job is not to understand foreign culture but to understand our own. Organizational culture is something which profoundly affects our action and yet is largely hidden from us – attending to this gives us the chance to stand back and reappraise aspects of our working world which we have become so used to that we take for granted ... in looking at culture it is vital to consider what is happening now before concentrating on what should happen in the future.

One model of organizational culture I like is that developed by Roger Harrison (1993), initially with Charles Handy (1976), who presents an uncomplicated view of how an organization can become oriented towards one of four basic cultural types as shown in Fig. 3.7.

POWER Culture:	ROLE Culture:
based on STRENGTH	based on STRUCTURE
* Direction * Decisiveness * Determination	* Order * Stability * Control
ACHIEVEMENT Culture:	SUPPORT Culture:
based on COMPETENCE	based on RELATIONSHIPS
* Growth * Success * Distinction	* Mutuality * Service * Integration

Fig. 3.7 Harrison's four organizational cultures (1993).

I see this framework as a way of getting an idea of the relative weighting an organization gives to these different orientations. It is intended as a way of describing the culture where you are, rather than as a means of making a good or bad judgement of it. Each of the four cultural types have their positive and negative sides and it is unlikely that any organization will exclusively fit any single type to the extreme. More often there is a mix of types that can be seen to be prominent and these will vary from organization to organization (and possibly from department to department within the same organization).

The model gives you a chance to identify the predominant orientation(s) where you work and to consider the advantages and pitfalls of each type. Figure 3.8 is an overview of the positives and negatives of each type. Make a note of those features that seem to relate to your organization as you read it through.

functional aspects	dysfunctional aspects

Power [Strength] Culture:

strong charismatic leadership that gives clarity and purpose; loyalty rewarded and people protected; wise, benevolent active leadership; demanding but fair leadership; you get ahead by complying and putting leader's wishes before your own	give boss's wishes top priority even if interferes with important work; afraid to give bad news; leaders not questioned even when seen to be wrong; when those with power break the rules etc; when advancement follows loyalty and allegiance rather than competence

Role [Structure] Culture:

performance assessed against the written job criteria; rewarded for being reliable, dependable and playing by the rules; inefficiency and confusion reduced by clear objectives; defined authority and responsibility of jobs; variability of job performance reduced by defined job infrastructure	where rules blindly followed even when counter productive; unpreparedness to exercise any initiative or constructive thought outside laid down procedures; more important not to be different than to do the right thing; individuality squeezed out; people treated as pieces of interchangeable equipment not people

Achievement [Competence] Culture:

where shared sense of urgency in achieving valued goals; sense of meaning and purpose; strong sense of self esteem; people voluntarily manage themselves; rules are not allowed to get in the way; high morale and cohesion; feeling of being part of something special	work becomes so important it takes over a person's life; belief becomes so strong that the ends justify the means; inward looking workings; competitive and arrogance tendencies increase; internal dissent and criticism stifled; begins to lose touch with those outside the group or organisation

Support [Relationships] Culture:

high level of mutual support and co-operation; harmony is valued and conflict resolution seen as a priority; being seen and valued as an individual important; strong sense of belonging and pleasure in being together	relationships may be focused on too much and the work neglected; difficult personnel issues may be ducked; scope for surface harmony but covert conflict; may lose direction and cohesion when consensus lost; comfy, complacence and ineffectiveness may arise; equal valuing may frustrate the more competent

Fig. 3.8 Overview of positive and negative aspects of each type.

Each of the types has beneficial qualities for an organization. The difficulty however is achieving a suitable balance between the pulls of each type as each type, in the extreme, has limitations that can ruin the whole organization.

If you look at your own organization which of the types is it

- most similar to,
- which would be the next most similar type,
- which do you see it as being least like?

When you look at your responses how would you then summarize your organization in words (see Fig. 3.9)?

If you can complete Fig. 3.9, you have another way of understanding your organization. You have even more insight into how you see and make sense of your organization. You can speculate more knowledgeably about why some matters seem more important than others and you have more chance of appreciating the impact it has (both positive and negative) on you and your work. For example:

- how displays of strong leadership can outweigh everything else in a power culture,
- how doing your job strictly as defined is accorded great importance in a *role*-oriented organization whereas,
- how committing yourself wholly to getting the job done, whatever the personal cost, is looked for and rewarded in an *achievement* culture, and
- where harmony, cohesion and positive morale are the tops in a support culture.

(i) I see my organisation as most like the .... culture

because ....(include both strengths and limitations of

the type as appropriate) ....

(ii) In addition I also see similarities with a number of the

characteristics of the .....(next most similar type, again cover

the strengths and limitations you see).... culture in that ....

(iii) My organisation however seems least like the .... type(s)

because .... and what this means here is that ....

Fig. 3.9   Describing my organization.

The effect of these preferences is that they can take over and influence the whole style, nature and tone of the organization. They become the predominant culture of that organization, possibly with disastrous effects so far as the effectiveness of that organization is concerned.

If you now re-read the description of your organization, check to what extent your organization has gone too far in emphasizing any one of these four styles at the expense of the others. Also, see if you can identify any of the main limitations noted in Fig. 3.8.You may want to test your assessment with colleagues but make sure they say what they think first, and then compare the responses.

Several writers have been exploring organizational culture in the past few years. References and further reading are available at the end of this chapter. You may prefer to use Harrison's approach (Harrison, 1993), or indeed put together some of your own ideas, before digging too deeply into other models. The key point is to see if through using the notion of organizational culture you can arrive at a more informed view of your organization and how it works.

Pulling these ideas and reflections together

You now have:

- the initial diagnosis you put together (see Fig. 3.1) resulting from the questions you asked yourself about your organization,
- three examples of how organizations can be looked at and set up,
- some ideas about the formal and informal organization,
- some ideas about organizational culture.

You can apply these ideas to any place you are working and they will enable you begin to answer some of the confusions and questions you may have about how those organizations are functioning.

Do remember that at any one time there are a number of different and competing perceptions of your organization in the minds of you and your colleagues. If you talk about the hospital, ward, clinic etc., as an organization your colleagues could be responding with one or more of the definitions as shown in Fig. 3.10.

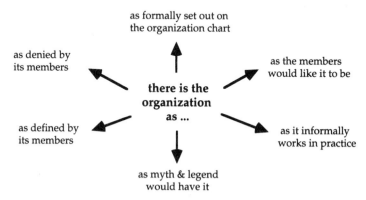

Fig. 3.10   Differing definitions of the organization.

Early in this chapter I posed two questions you may want to ask about your experience of being in an organization. The first was 'How can this be...?' and the second was 'Are we unusual in this as an organization?'. You now have several perspectives about the nature, make-up and internal workings of organizations that you can use to form your own response to these two questions. By applying these ideas to your own organization(s) you can begin to understand them better.

Why all this matters

The organizational models outlined can be used to diagnose what is going on around you and to build up an idea of just how well your organization is functioning. With so much of your career likely to be spent in one organization or another the ideas covered here may help you to identify the types and styles of organization you prefer. These ideas will also – together with those in Part Four – help you to play your part in facilitating constructive change.

The culture of an organization will affect how you can do your professional work, the quality of the relationships you have with your colleagues and the degree to which you can be yourself in doing your work in a careful and professional manner. Understanding the culture is an important skill.

Part One has set out the contexts in which you operate as a nurse and drawn attention to some of the underlying personal and institutional dynamics that will influence your clinical practice. Part Two moves the focus of attention from the settings in which you work onto *you* in all this.

References

Braten, S. (1983) Hvor gar grensen for bedriftslokale kulturer? Hoel, M. and Hvinden, B. (ned) *Kollectivteori og Sosiologi.* Glydendal, Oslo.

Hall, E. (1959) *The Silent Language* Doubleday, New York.

Handy, C. (1976) *Understanding Organizations* Penguin Books, Harmondsworth.

Harrison, R. (1993) *Diagnosing Organizational Culture*, Pfeiffer and Co. San Diego, USA.

Galbraith, J.W. (1977) *Organizational Design*, Addison-Wesley, Reading, MA.

McLean, A. and Marshall, J. (1983) *Intervening in Cultures*, University of Bath.

Ouchi, W. and Johnson, J. (1978) Types of organizational control and their relationship to emotional well-being. *Administrative Science Quarterly*, **23**, pp 292–317.

Peters, T. and Waterman, R. (1982) *In Search of Excellence* Harper and Row, New York.

Van Maanen, J. and Schein, E. (1988) in *Cultures at Work*, Local Government Training Board, Luton.

Weisbord, M. (1978) *Organizational Diagnosis* Addison-Wesley, Reading, USA.

Wilkins, A. (1983) Organizational stories as symbols which control the organization, in Pondy, L. (eds) *Organizational Symbolism*, Greenwich, Ct. JAI.

Further reading

Deal, T. and Kennedy, A. (1982) *Corporate Cultures* Addison-Wesley, Reading, USA.

Hampden-Turner, C. (1990) *Corporate Culture for Competitive Edge* Economist Publications, London.

McKenna, E. (1994) *Business Psychology and Organisational Behaviour*, Lawrence Erlbaum Associates Ltd, Hove.

McLean, A. and Marshall, J. (1988) *Cultures at Work*, Local Government Training Board, Luton.

Morgan, G. (1986) *Images of Organization* Sage Publications, London.

PART TWO:
REFLECTIONS, REVIEW AND REVELATIONS

This part moves the focus from the organizational to the personal: to *you* in it all. Initially inviting you to clarify the views you have of yourself, before looking at where you are in relation to the various stages of life we pass through. Chapter 6 suggests ways of using these ideas further.

While I think it unlikely that, at the end of this chapter, you will suddenly say 'Yes, that's it: that is me!' you will be able to do quite a lot in sketching out who you see yourself to be, and perhaps what you seek to achieve in life. There are several advantages of doing this type of reflection:

- to be clearer about what is important to you,
- to generate more belief in yourself,
- for clarity about what to value, change and develop,
- for a broader perspective on life,
- for more inner knowledge, balance and ease.

While my focus is on you as a nurse I see the material we are looking at as providing ideas and perspectives that these you can apply more generally whatever you are engaged in to help you navigate yourself through your life.

Chapter 4
Who Am I and Where Am I Going?

It was a 39 year old senior manager's birthday. He usually woke each day with a
tightness in his stomach and found it difficult to relax even when off duty.
'What would you like for your birthday?' his wife asked.
'What about peace, kindness to all men . . . peace of mind . . .' he replied.
'I was thinking about a jumper' she said.

Who am I (and why does it matter)?

While this may seem a strange, or even an unnecessary question, it
really is a crucially important one. Building up your sense of who and
what you are is one of the most important pieces of work you can do. I
am not suggesting you sit and look at the mirror and repeat the question
over and over again until 'the answer' comes to you in a blinding flash of
insight. However, it is something that is on people's minds more often
than we may realize. As it is so important, you may like to set aside some
time to reflect on how you see yourself. You don't necessarily need to do
this now but as you go through the book and begin to apply the ideas
you will be missing a great deal if you don't, at the same time, begin to
sketch in more about yourself. Your reflections need to cover both those
attributes you like to see and those aspects that you find less appealing.
All the different aspects of you are important to acknowledge.

One method of doing this is to give yourself some quiet time and
reflect on how you see yourself. Let thoughts float into your mind and
make a few notes. Think back on your memories and let the thoughts,
questions, confusions, settings, colours, ideas and feelings and emotions
etc., emerge. Make some notes of the things which seem important to
you otherwise you may forget them. In my experience doing this takes
time, and different things come into your mind at different times. Also
your views, recollections and feelings alter as you go along. Over a
period of time you will be able to compile a collection of facets and
aspects that you consider accurately describe important aspects of your
self.

You should make a start soon, because you will get more out of this
book if you can. Whatever notes you make you will want to come back
to them later to add in more material and look again at what you put

down previously. As this process goes on you will see things a little differently. This process of seeing how your perceptions alter about yourself is both a revealing and thought provoking one.

There are a few prompts in Fig. 4.1 to help you make a start. Please pull these thoughts together into a description (see Fig. 4.2) because you will then be able to draw on these initial thoughts as you go through the chapter.

Thoughts	Accomplishments	Doubts
Strengths	Weaknesses	Successes
Failures	Pleasures	Vices
Virtues	Sexuality	Physical form
Wants	Needs	Dreams etc

Fig. 4.1 Building up a picture of myself.

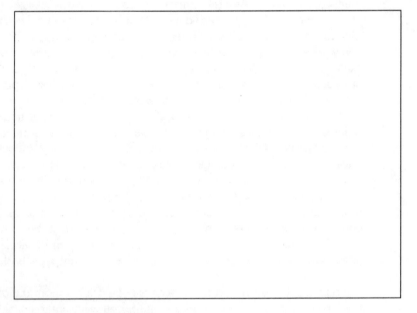

Fig. 4.2 Initial description of me as I see myself.

Often we are told *who* or *what* we are by others, and often most of us seem prepared to accept others' views of us and we carry them with us for many years. This can be very frustrating and constraining – as well as inaccurate. Only we can know who we are and what we feel. All too rarely we try to work out who we are for ourselves or challenge what others are telling us about ourselves. This can have a devastating effect on a person's image of himself. They are put down by others and so begin to have less self-regard and self-belief, or else they may be held in such high esteem that they get caught up in trying to meet unrealistic expectations of others.

Either way there are costs and dangers. While we do not live unaffected by the views others have of us, the more realistic a view we have of ourselves the more likely we will be able to learn fully from our experiences. It is very easy to get trapped into this type of good/bad thinking, where we allow our self-belief to become dependent on the outcome of events over which we have limited influence.

What may be more fruitful is

- To acknowledge both positive and negative experiences as valid information to take account of.
- Not to see them as either good or bad statements about your worth as a person.
- To be able to learn from what occurred for next time.

If you can combine your assessment of what went on with what you know about yourself (self-knowledge), you will be able to learn from the experience and do better next time rather than feeling vulnerable and at the mercy of what is going on around you.

However, being able to acknowledge and learn from your successes and disappointments is neither straightforward nor easy. It means that you have to be able to own up to yourself about what is going on. You need to feel secure enough to admit negative information about yourself; to learn to accept criticism without falling apart.

Whilst there is a need to protect oneself from harm – psychological as well as physical – this is not helped by rejecting relevant accurate data you may prefer not to acknowledge. By building up your own knowledge of, and belief in, yourself you can become more resilient in the face of adversity, threat and disappointment than you were before.

Clarifying how you see yourself helps you to be clearer and more confident about what you do and don't want, and about what you are looking for in the future. It can enable you to look at the past from a more intergrated personal perspective.

One thing to remember is that your perspective on matters and past experiences will alter as you go through life – and however subjective – it can be very enlightening to see the way your views of yourself differed over time. So you may want to keep the notes and reflections you make; date them for future reference.

Most of us have 'blind spots' and things we can't – or are not prepared – to see or wish to acknowledge about ourselves but which are noticed by others. One means of finding more out about these blind spots is to build up the quality of your relationships and to encourage others to feed back to you some of those aspects of yourself that you were not aware of.

A method for going about this called the Johari window is explained in Chapter 8. However, for the moment continue to build up your view of yourself by noting down in Fig. 4.3 what you know about yourself and what others have told you.

What I'm told   ... ..and.....   **What I know**

:

:

:

:

Fig. 4.3   What I have been told about myself.

In addition to these notes there will be aspects of you of which you are unaware (an out-of-awareness segment) and material that you may never be able to access (the unconscious). There will also be aspects of you that you see as part of you and don't want to acknowledge because they are difficult to accept or downright distasteful.

All of us, I suspect, have a darker side containing those aspects which can frighten us and which contain negative, hateful, aggressive and unpalatable drives, feelings and motivations. A side to our humanity which seems to be driven by destructive instincts and needs that is contrary to our upbringing. We anticipate that these instincts would be shocking to others if they knew about them.

As these 'other sides' co-exist with the more socially acceptable parts of us, rather than seeking to repress, deny or run away from them, it may be more constructive to acknowledge them. Where you consider it helpful, share some of these less appealing thoughts you have from time to time with others. You may be surprised to find that some of your darker and hidden thoughts and feelings, confusions and fantasies may be similar to those held by others. This may help you to come to terms with them as a part of you, and help you to put them into perspective. They do not necessarily mean that you are abnormal, an outcast or strange – nor that you will be impelled to act on them.

Occasionally sharing some of this material may enable you to develop a more rounded view of yourself, and the world. It will show you that there is a mix of the good and the bad *and* that they co-exist and contain within each the seeds of the other. Denying the existence, or the potential, for the darker side of our nature paradoxically increases the chance that these destructive facets of human nature may suddenly emerge and take us by surprise. Always emphasizing the positive, for example, denies the possibility of manipulative undertones that can underpin the expressed good intentions.

Figure 4.4 highlights several more questions which – if you answer them as fully as you can – will help you to build up a fuller picture of how you see yourself. View your responses as if they are a set of working hypotheses about you. You can then test them over the coming days and weeks, and revise them in the light of your experiences and your further reflections. The great value is that it will help you to become more secure and knowledgeable about who you are and what matters to you.

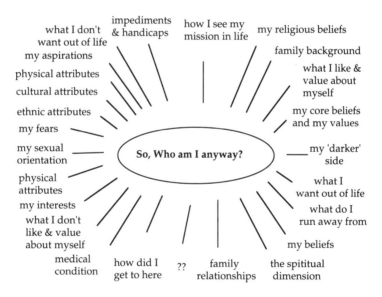

Fig. 4.4 Building up a picture of me.

There is a lot of material in this figure so take it a piece at a time, and you may want to add in some additional dimensions. My purpose in asking you to think about these matters is that it will help you become clearer about:

- what matters to you,
- what you shut out,

- what you stand up for and
- what you are not at all interested in, etc.

Over time, by working through these questions, and aspects of your life, you will begin to get closer to describing yourself. Your descriptions are not the complete story. Others have information about you too and they will see and know things about you that you don't. You will need to tap into these other sources in due course. However, just by listening carefully and watching what is going on will tell you a great deal too about how you are regarded and about the impact you make.

The format in Fig. 4.5 is one you could use to record your data and help you to organize it for future use.

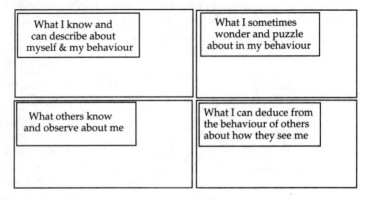

Fig. 4.5   Reflections on myself.

How you 'show' yourself and how others see you?

It is one thing to make your own notes about yourself but at some stage these will need to be supplemented by the views and perspectives from those around you. They have their own view of who and what you are to them and they will see and experience you differently. The process of pulling all these pieces of information together, and of checking them to see what sense you can make of them, will enable you to construct a more integrated view of who you are.

You are on 'show' every time you are in the view of others. I say this not to make you preoccupied with this fact – or to make you overly self-conscious – but to emphasize the point that those around you have a great deal of data on you *and* that you too have an enormous amount of information about yourself to draw upon. Usually, however, these banks of data do not get drawn on or used in an ordered way. You need to consciously take notice of how and to what, you find yourself reacting to as you go about things.

My aim is to encourage you to operate on more than one level of experiencing what is going on – both in and around you – at the same time. By deliberately noticing what you are doing and the reactions you are receiving, as an observer of yourself-in-action, you will be more able to understand, make sense of and cope with the situations that you have to deal with. By reflecting on these interactive processes more consciously you can pick up much about what you actually do as opposed to what you may say, or think, you do.

In many ways we actively project how we want others to see us. We do this when we decide what to wear, how to act when in the company of others, where we go, what and how we say things, and in the opinions and beliefs we express. When we look at another person we begin to sum them up, based on our experiences of them, on what we see, from our imagination and from the assumptions we draw from all these clues given us by the other person. We will notice many things: colours of their clothes, hairstyle, choice of adornments, gait and physical style of movement, speech patterns etc. We will use this data to form assumptions about who they are, what they do and what they may believe in.

You do this all the time too. Think back to the ward or clinic when you see a new patient or client for the first time. It is often difficult *not* to sum them up even before you have listened to much of their history, their condition, their needs etc. We automatically do it. Part of your developing skill will be to slow down your ability to process and categorize the person in front of you and to give them the chance to tell you about themselves. Give them the opportunity to challenge the unstated assumptions you may have. At the same time, holding back your personal assessment will only be productive if you listen to them carefully and attentively. Only then will you be in a position to come to some tentative conclusions about who they are and what they may be like.

Each of us has a choice in how we show ourselves to the world. It is something we give extensive thought to. Even when uniforms are worn it is surprising how we can still contrive to present a persona for ourselves that differentiates us from our colleagues. We look for acceptable ways which will make it easier for us to be perceived as different from the nurse next to us. This is seen on the ward, both in our static physical presentation and through our movement and deportment about the ward or in the clinic.

It is how we choose to put together our physical, emotional, social and intellectual background that makes us unique. Even if the two of us were to experience the same event, and even if we agreed on the critical incidents and the progress of events, the sense and personal meaning we then each make of it *for ourselves* will be different. If from what can be observed, recorded and heard we may be of one mind, there will still be differences in the meaning and importance we attribute to that event and of our experience of it.

Precisely how we integrate the personal impacts of our experiences with our knowledge, and how we derive meaning from these is very personal. One could say it is a *unique* process which no one else can possibly do or replicate. While there are many facets of us that are commonly shared with others we have to be different because no one else can have exactly the same experience of life.

Figure 4.6 identifies some of the ways in which we show aspects of who we are and what we want to be seen or experienced as by others. We can, however, only exercise choice over some of these dimensions.

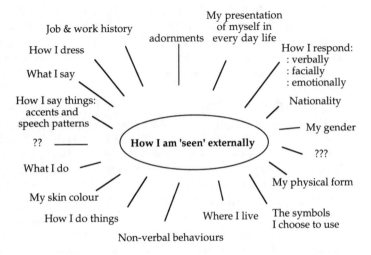

Fig. 4.6   How I 'show' myself.

Many of these facets reflect the external persona of a person. While these are very influential in creating initial impressions, they reveal little about the deeper self of the person. Yet because a person has chosen to present in particular ways they do give us some inkling of what that person is about and how they might see themselves. This in turn will reflect that person's inner self.

In professional and business life there are expectations about how to present oneself which reflect the norms and expectations of that profession and business. The degree to which we are able (or choose) to meet such expectations will influence whether we are welcomed and accepted or frowned upon and possibly discounted by that community. In many ways we affect our future, and our standing in the eyes of others, by what we externally present ourselves as being. It is not surprising, therefore, that so much attention is given to the external presentation of self.

In nursing, there are strong peer group pressures and devices that, for sound clinical reasons perhaps, lead nurses to present themselves in a professionally conventional way. They are generally in uniform, with marks of seniority and of professional accomplishment prominently and proudly on display.

There is much about the profession that leads non-nurses to see nurses as being almost individually indistinguishable. It is as if they are all the same, and able to give the same degree of care and specialist expertise irrespective of the widely differing needs of the patient or client. Yet this is not the case. There are significant technical differences between the nursing specialities. These make it almost impossible – and dangerous – for any qualified nurse to be able to work at any nursing station without the necessary post-basic training.

The selection procedures, the professional training, and the socialization processes of nurse training result in colleagues who have a shared body of knowledge and best practice. They are able to deal with many traumatic and difficult situations. Their ethical training and propriety – together with the emotional bonding of the work – creates a bedrock of professional cohesion and sameness to the outside observer. It is part of the mystique and part of the protection of being a nurse.

To reach a fuller picture of any person (particularly a nurse in a uniform) will usually mean that you will have to look beyond what is formally presented. You will need to observe them and see how they are able to stamp their own individual mark on what they do, while meeting the social and professional expectations set for them.

As a nurse, you are expected to present yourself in ways that reflect your professional role, your personal standing in the profession and as a member of the care setting in which you are placed. There needs to be sufficient integration of these to demonstrate that you are a part of the team. At the same time there is you as yourself. You will want to show your individuality but you will not have complete freedom of choice to do so. It is likely that there will be some tension generated because of this conflict between what you are required to be and who you are.

This raises questions of power, control, independence, security, trust, rebellion and frustration among others. It will raise questions (see Fig. 4.7) about how this tension can be handled and mediated by you.

Your thoughts on questions such as these will give you even more information about who you are; the extent to which this shows itself and is displayed, or held back from those around you. An important question is can you be one person at work and a rather different one outside the nursing environment?

Is there one me – or several?

Often people talk about themselves as 'not being me', of 'not feeling myself today' or 'now, the real me can come out', or – in commenting

---

• How does all this work for you?

• Do you feel that you have choices and can make your own decisions or do you consider that the opportunities for choice open to you are very limited?

• To what degree do you feel able to show yourself as you would like to or do you find it better for you not to stand out at all from those around you?

• And if you do choose to stand out, in what ways do you do this and why do you think you made those particular choices?

Fig. 4.7 Handling the professional *v* personal pulls and tensions.

on somebody else – 'I don't know who the real *X* is '. It suggests that there is a single (and relatively consistent) self. However, while there is a central core, there are many 'me's' each of which shows itself depending on what is going on and the particular choices I have made in response to the current situation I am in.

As far as I am concerned, the notion of the 'self' is a multiple and not a single one. It is all *me*, what you see is a varying reflection (or representation) of me: but it is all the same me. This is my experience from reflections on myself, and of being with other people through various situations. I have seen them as very different at times, but nevertheless retaining their sense of self while responding to what is going on around and within them.

It also seems to me to be presumptuous of any person to try to tell someone else that they are being or not being themselves. Surely the only person who knows that is the person concerned. It cannot be anyone else even though someone else can know when I am less at ease with myself. Even then it is still 'me' even if it is one slightly out of tune.

For example, have you experienced situations where you were told you were not 'being normal', or not being 'yourself', or where you were told 'to be like' someone else? Certainly you can consider developing attributes that are seen in others as valuable, and to be emulated, if you choose to. In this case you will do it in your own way and bring all of your own experiences, biases, fears and accomplishments with you in the process.

One of the difficulties that can be experienced from time to time is when we wish that we could suddenly be like someone else. Yet it cannot happen for us unless we do it ourselves. No one else can change us from the inside except ourselves. Even then the result is (and can only be) a different us, not a replication of somebody else we have seen and wanted to be like.

What you choose to do in the presence of others matters to you, even if you feel you have let yourself down or, in some way, not come up to scratch, or if you say you don't care. How you present yourself in everyday life is equally important for those around you too, whether they be a patient, a doctor, or a visitor.

What about those aspects of ourselves that are not readily visible; the parts of us that we keep to ourselves; parts which are just as real, perhaps more so, than anything that can be seen or touched externally. This is what we will discuss in the next section.

The internal world of me

A point worth making is that you are special; you are complex and how and why you do things is hard to explain for much of the time. We may have been trained in logic, reason, analysis and scientific rigour yet however helpful and influential these processes may be, when it comes down to human behaviour a whole raft of additional influences come into play. These respond to a different, more emotively charged, set of logic other than a purely rational one. Our actions and thoughts will not necessarily be consistent, easy to predict or be based on what is tangible or readily explained to others.

It is similar to the process people follow when deciding to buy something such as a car. Have you ever gone through the business of comparing prices, the features on offer, the 'special deals', the warranty arrangements, miles per gallon, depreciation rates, insurance costs, the 'cashback' offers . . . and so on. You actually made your mind up right at the start *yet* went through all this logical–rational stuff because others expected you to do so, or because you thought you ought to. However your predisposition though only gets exposed on those occasions when, having done all the comparisons, the choice you wanted all along does not show up as either the first or second choice (or best buy). Yet you buy it anyway, against the analysis you have carefully completed! This can leave those around you a bit confused (and amused or exasperated or angry) about your behaviour and they may say 'Look, if you wanted to buy the Jag anyway, why did you go through all the pointless analysis?'. Why indeed?

We are a bit like this in our behaviour. We may have been trained to function in a logical manner but find that we also function in ways that surprise, sometimes confound and certainly (with hindsight) we might find confusing. This suggests that in addition to the criteria we say we are following – as with the example of selecting a car – we are also following additional influences that are less visible or apparent.

One way of thinking about ourselves and what makes us as we are is to view ourselves as if we had several layers of understanding and of meaning – as with the onion skin diagram (Fig. 1.3). At the very heart of us are those aspects that lie deep down and determine who we are and what makes us 'tick'. They are the deepest and the most private parts of us and they will be protected and strongly defended should they come under threat. They shape and drive the meanings we give to our experiences and because they are at the centre of things they are held dear.

So much of us is derived from these inner aspects that they are very difficult to change. Genuine, fundamental change at this level of the person comes from inside rather than through the imposition of external pressures. At times I know I have had to do things, or go along with a situation, that I initially resisted because it was the only option. But this was a superficial change when under a threat. Deep down there was no change at all and I maintained my core beliefs even though what was observed in my behaviour could have suggested to some that I had changed.

In Fig. 4.8 I have shown these core perspectives and determinants at the centre of the diagram. You have to 'peel back', as with an onion, or cut through everything else first before you can get to the core of anyone. Then at the core are the values, the beliefs, the attitudes and the fears that determine our external reactions and behaviours. The contents of this centre area could be said to be the essence of us and – not surprisingly – these parts of us will be very strongly protected and held close by us.

Our core beliefs are our source of inner regard, strength and cohesion, and these will drive a person to tackle many situations and guide them in how they take action and respond to external events. While to

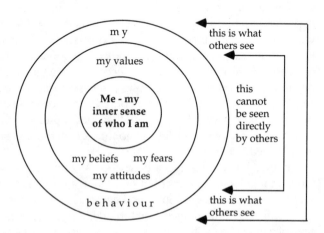

Fig. 4.8 Core beliefs.

others our actions may, at times, appear unexpected or unusual, there will be, even in cases of mental distress, some internal logic and rationale, guiding our behaviour. The key to understanding ourselves, and others, is to begin to understand the many varying considerations influencing our thinking and understanding that are centred in this core part of ourselves.

We are by no means geared up to work and make decisions only on the basis of a scientific rational–logical approach, because at the same time we are subject and respond to less rational impulses, drives and wishes. What seems important is not to try to cast everything into a logical–rational format but to begin to acknowledge and understand the non logical–rational ways of working that we are all subject to. The logic may be located in some of our more deeply held beliefs, or they may be unknown to us, in our unconscious perhaps. But they exist and they exert a strong influence on what we feel and what we do.

We are all a bit of a mix – no matter how we seek to present ourselves, and no matter how we see it from the inside – of constructive and destructive instincts and impulses. We are also continually struggling to put all of this together for ourselves in a way that makes sense to us and which enables us to remain functional as people in a social world; and this can be difficult to achieve at times.

There are some things we will be relatively clear about. For example, why we do things in a particular way or why we just 'don't like' doing something else. These may be related to difficult (or pleasurable) past experiences or they could be associated with some self doubts and fears in us. In some cases we may be able to acknowledge to ourselves some of the internal dynamics and issues that lead us to avoid particular situations or to respond in ways which may to others seem unexpected, unhelpful or unusual. Of course other people will be unaware of how we see it from our internal perspective and they will not know about our past experiences.

It may be helpful to keep in mind when you are caring for a patient, and when you are with a colleague, that we all have our own issues to work with. While you will know some of them, there will be some of which you will remain unaware even though they will affect you and influence what you do. It will be the same too for your patients and your colleagues.

These thoughts can be taken in several ways:

- They can be dismissed as rubbish. What you can't see does not exist and anyway it doesn't affect me. What is this business of 'the inside me' anyway?
- You may think that there is a lot about me that others don't know. They shouldn't anyway, because what would they think of me then? I wish he wouldn't write about these things; it's easier just getting on with the job isn't it?

- It could be that these ideas begin to open up and make more sense of some things that have been troubling or perplexing you over the years. The response may be, 'Um well that *is* interesting because I do know that how I show myself is not always an accurate reflection of who I am but that is what is expected from me isn't it?' I realize that I still have to work on and take more account of, the inside parts of me and I think that working with these ideas is something worthwhile.

I don't know if any of these three reactions reflect your thoughts but it is worthwhile checking out your reactions and making a few brief notes – see Fig. 4.9. You may find it helpful to see in black and white what your views are now about this material; they may also alter as time goes on.

---

1. They do not make sense because ...

2. Yes, they are helping me to make some connections because ...

3. Look, let's leave well enough alone and just concentrate on the job OK, because ...

Fig. 4.9   My initial reactions to these ideas.

Much of what goes on within us is reflected in our thoughts about who we are, how competent we see ourselves and in the self monitoring conversations we hold that tell us what we should or should not be doing. What we think, what we imagine and what we believe are powerful and critical influences on our behaviour and our state of psychological well-being.

Systems of belief and meaning : our audio and video tapes

We have very fertile minds and a tremendous capacity for imagination. We can create options and possibilities that no one has spelt out in detail to us, yet we can create them nevertheless. We have an ability to replay (not always with complete accuracy though) past situations. We are able to reflect and reconsider what went on and – *this is really important* – what might be in the future. We can make assumptions and we can predict.

We can use and apply these great abilities for good and ill; to help and to hinder us. We can take a situation and make it positive and developmental, and we can take a similar (maybe even the same) situation and see it as depressive, negative and demeaning. From the first interpretation we emerge more engaged and robust, whereas from the second interpretation we emerge as self-doubting, flawed and with a sense of failure.

We make sense of what we experience on the basis of past behaviour, learning from significant others and critical events. We make judged assessments about the future and we have some inherited predispositions that are also part of our make-up. The assumptions we make about ourselves and others impact significantly on our subsequent personal interactions. We then internalize – as standards of practice for ourselves – those patterns of behaviour that we have successfully predicted and anticipated. We build up our own system of belief and meaning that makes sense to us.

These thinking and checking-out processes go on largely unnoticed, but all the time we are processing what we see going on. We make the best sense of it that we can given the frameworks of personal meaning we have constructed for ourselves. Since much of this goes on unnoticed – in the same way that paint dries, or wood warps – it is very possible that we may continue to base our behaviour and beliefs on, what has now become, inappropriate or irrelevant data from the past.

Beck (1976) reports, for example, how he found that patients had to be trained to recall what thoughts they had prior to unpleasant feelings or sensations. These 'automatic thoughts' would pass by almost unnoticed – unless specifically asked for. Either patients were not fully conscious of them or it did not occur to them that these thoughts warranted special scrutiny. They accepted their current experiences and did not consider a different outcome as a possibility. He considered that

> ... the content of people's internal signals or automatic thoughts are shaped by their rules. People possess *mental rule books* to guide their actions and to evaluate themselves and others. These rules are absorbed to a large extent through observation of others and through personal experience. Once detected, the rules, and the evaluative inferences drawn from them can help explain seemingly illogical behaviours and irrational emotional responses.

Kelly's 'personal constructs' (1955), Meichenbaum's 'internal dialogues' (1977), Beck's 'mental rule books' (1976), Ellis's 'rational and irrational thinking' patterns (1973), together with Brewin and Antaki's (1987) work on categories of 'individual attribution of meaning' – record and catalogue some of the ways in which the individual seeks to weave together their own systems of meaning and belief based on their accumulated experiences.

These cognitive approaches suggest that each individual constructs their own sets of understandings about themself in-the-world. Also that each individual will have their own way of organizing and making sense of their experiences.

It may be that, as Lane (1989) suggests 'unless we believe something we do not see it' and it may also be that unless we know how to look at something we are unclear as to what it is and what it means for us. Ellis comments

> ... that people seem so easily conditioned into dysfunctional thinking and behaviour and also that [as] this is so hard to modify, ... [it is] ... evidence of an innate tendency to irrationality. People's failure to think rationally and face reality almost always leads them to manifest the feelings and behaviours of emotional disturbance. (Ellis, 1973.)

This suggests that not only do we create our own understandings of what life is all about *but* also that we can get trapped into unhelpful thinking patterns. These constrain and limit what we think we can do and consequently what we try to do!

Some suggest that we pack all these thoughts, experiences, pressures, into a format that gives us a guide as to what we can and cannot do depending on the issue, the dynamics involved, the setting and our sense of ourselves in relation to all of this. Beck's (1976) view is that these automatic thoughts and internal signals that we give ourselves are shaped by the rules we have laid down.

In various ways this book invites *you* to make more obvious and apparent to yourself the contents of the 'rule book' you have constructed and work from. Once detected, you can identify the rules you follow; speculate on where they may have originated and the impact they have on your thinking and behaviour. This can help you to explain, and throw more light on, some of the seemingly illogical behaviours and responses that you realize you have been making.

Ellis considers that:

> For all practical purposes, the sentences that people keep saying to themselves are or become their thoughts and emotions. Thus people's self-statements are capable of both generating and modifying their emotions – so people re-indoctrinate themselves with irrational thinking and faulty self-statements. In this respect, human beings largely control their own destinies through innate, acquired and continuously re-indoctrinated beliefs they hold or of how they believe things will occur. People's beliefs can be either rational and functional or irrational and self defeating.

This is an important notion, that what you say to yourself is 'capable of both generating and modifying' your behaviour. In many ways, what you believe about yourself will affect what you subsequently feel able or not able to do.

If this is so significant, a key to understanding a person pivots around helping them to be clearerer about their internal discussions and debates. Also, what meaning they take from their private conversations. Meichenbaum (1977) uses the term 'internal dialogue' to describe these internal discussions about meanings, where we have a process of both listening and talking to oneself in a self-communication system. But how does all this happen and what does this mean for you?

How you think about matters affects who you are and what you do

What we mull over in the conversations we have with ourselves from time to time can influence what we can and cannot do. If we believe we can't be the student representative, or represent the clinic at a conference, then we will find it hard to carry out that task if we are forced to. At the same time if we have internal dialogues about belief in what we can do, it may be more likely that this will happen. The more you can make a note of the internal conversations, the clearer you will become about how you are conditioning yourself for future performance.

Note in particular any negative self-talk you realize you are engaging in. This is likely to be adversely affecting your well-being. For example, where you tell yourself that you can't do something, or that you are not any good at something. It may have begun years back when you didn't do well but were told by somebody that you would *never* be any good at that: and you believed them!

The creation of your own rule book comes from various sources; the most significant are probably:

- what you have been told about yourself over the years (good, bad, bright, stupid, artistic, creative, strong, will be successful, destructive, unworthy, a born leader),
- how you have been treated (your experience of life, the reactions you have received from others, what you have seen others doing etc.).

You then slowly put this together and you will have your own personal manual of what you are about, how you are valued and what you have found you need to survive and get on in life. All the time you are updating your rule book based on your current experiences but there are two main barriers that can skew this updating process. First you are likely to disregard data if it challenges your current thinking patterns. For example, if you did something rather well that your internal thinking predicted you would be no good at, you may disregard the good outcome as luck or a fluke. Second, you will tend not to do those things – unless you can't avoid them – that you don't think you can do or are any good at. You therefore don't give yourself opportunities to practise and become more accomplished at such tasks.

So, there are some in-built mental blocks that make it quite hard for you to change or challenge your negative beliefs. Unless you become quite rigorous in noting what these are and deliberately challenging them, you will not break out of the negative cycle.

Where do we start? Here are some thoughts to consider:

- You have your lifetime's worth of data to support your view of what is possible for you and what seems less possible.
- You have your own internal audio tape collection which provides internal commentaries on how you are, what you are doing, how to respond, what not to do, what to watch out for, what you cannot do – and have failed at in the past – what to guard against etc.
- You have your personal frameworks of meaning that enable you to make 'sense' of the world around you, and of your place within it.

Not much of this is obvious or readily apparent however. You may need to do some work on identifying what you know of the above and noticing more precisely what you do, what you are thinking etc.

These internal messages both reinforce and lead you to continue to play out your current story lines and the roles set out for you as if they are fixed for ever and 'the truth'. So far as a person's internal world is concerned there is no finite truth. Only so much is accessible and in thinking back to past events and experiences memories fade and change. We may think we remember everything, but we may not be quite as accurate as we would like to think we are. Most of us put a rosy gloss on aspects of our lives that were less positive than we now present them to be. Sometimes it serves a need to exaggerate both the good and the bad but there is no objective truth so far as our background is concerned. Our perspectives and understandings also change over time and lead us to see things differently, and perhaps to see them more clearly for what they were.

However, the internal messages and stories exert a tremendous effect on each of us:

- they can lead us to limit our horizons unnecessarily,
- they can lead us to become less able to do things that are perfectly within the scope of what we could accomplish,
- they can lead us to hold an unrealistically strong belief in our ability beyond our capabilities.

Whether the messages are too limiting or too ambitious we will come to believe them and act accordingly. These beliefs, and consequently the behaviour they generate, will influence how we see things, how we present ourselves to others and, critically, our sense of personal well-being.

Your view of what you can and cannot do is affected by whether or not internally you are telling yourself you can or cannot do certain things. By being very clear about the internal dialogues you can reconsider what is important. At the same time you are susceptible to what others say about you – positive and negative. If things are said often enough or loudly enough, you can begin to believe them, even if there is no basis to the assertions being made.

You may find it helpful to stop reading now and think about these ideas of internal dialogues and 'rule books' to decide if they make any sense to you. You may like to use Fig. 4.10 to start making a note of the internalized messages you give yourself, and some of the views of yourself you hear from others.

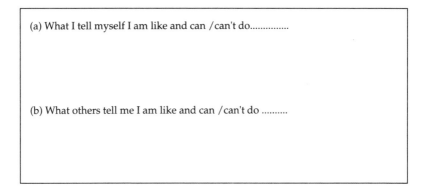

(a) What I tell myself I am like and can / can't do..............

(b) What others tell me I am like and can / can't do ....

Fig. 4.10 My internal messages and those from others.

Try to recall as many of these internal messages as you can. It is likely these will be constraining and influencing your behaviour and because the messages are now so familiar you may not readily notice what is happening. You may not like to accept that there is a possibility of these things happening. It is worth considering this possibility, and to make a note of any negative thinking about your potential, your capabilities or your performance that come to mind.

Now look at the list item by item and try to clarify:

- why it is there and where it came from,
- if you believe it is accurate or still the case,
- decide what you want to do about it, if anything.

It is likely that there are some messages that are no longer accurate descriptions of you and need to be let go. You may have realized that there are people who are continuing to tell you, inappropriately, what you are like, and/or what you are capable of doing or not doing. They will, at some stage, need to be told that their view is no longer accurate. Also you may have identified situations or responsibilities that you now feel you can handle with sufficient confidence that hitherto you have avoided, so look for an appropriate opportunity to start doing those things.

Negative thinking spirals

One way of thinking about these processes of negative thinking is to see them as a spiral that becomes harder and harder to break out of the more it persists. Figure 4.11 illustrates how it can operate using public speaking as the example.

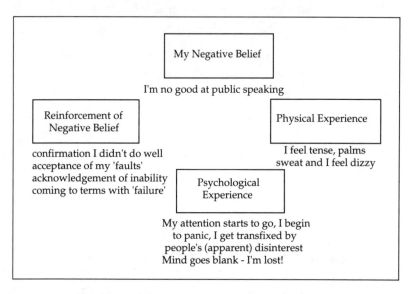

Fig. 4.11   A negative thinking spiral.

The person carries into their presentation a belief that they are no good at public speaking. They become acutely aware of signs of physical distress which they attribute to their negative belief. They forget that most people have some degree of anxiety and physical response in such situations and this carries over to their psychological experience. They are so convinced they are unable to do this that they interpret audience movement as an indictment of their inability. They begin to panic, lose their way in the presentation and – not surprisingly – it does falter. Finally, the feedback confirms their worst fears: they are no good!

Now the decision you have to make, having clarified for yourself what is happening, is if you want to break this negative pattern. In the example in Fig. 4.11 does the person want to improve their public speaking? It may seem a pointless question. But, the negative belief came about because in some way it suited you to adopt that belief. If the answer is a wish to change things then the next decision is to decide *how* to do that.

In Fig. 4.12 I have suggested some antidotes to each stage of the spiral outlined in Fig. 4.11. You can begin breaking out of this pattern at any of these points, and eventually you will cover all four of the points mentioned.

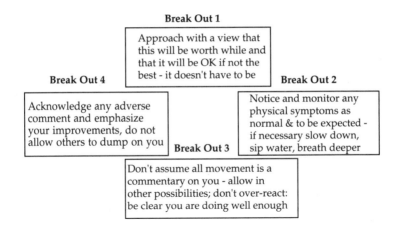

Fig. 4.12 Breaking out of the spiral.

Working from the examples in Fig. 4.12 above, select one of your own negative patterns and build up a similar diagram to Fig. 4.11 and describe it as completely as you can. Then you can move to the break-out diagram of Fig. 4.12 and decide on your own strategy for breaking out depending on the details of your own example. Take things at the speed that your judgement tells you is most appropriate. By identifying what you want to work on as a significant achievement, be strategic in planning your campaign to change things.

The thinking patterns we have led ourselves to believe in are not the final position on the matter. As Fig. 4.12 indicates, there are ways of breaking out of them if needs be. You can now explore the way that suits you best to break these negative cycles of thinking about yourself and to replace them with a more equally balanced perspective. Accept that you may experience difficulties in doing certain things but that you can improve, should you choose to.

Making a change to an established pattern will be hard. So much of what we do has a purpose that makes sense to us at some level. This could be because it meets some (stated or unstated) needs we have. It may defend us from a real or perceived threat; or fit in with what is expected of us by others and which suits us at that time. Changing this type of personal protection is therefore a risky business and needs to be taken with care.

Insights and taking action

This chapter began by asking you to trace and record things about yourself as part of the task of starting to define who you are and what is important to you. Some of this was probably quite easy to identify and record whereas other aspects may have left you wondering. The key is to start thinking about yourself in a way that will enable you to build up a more complete and constructive picture of who you are, what you do and what you can do more fully in the future.

It can be surprising how often other people are more sensitive to our inner selves. They can pinpoint things that we have been unable to see. You may be surprised at how accurately someone else can describe your feelings that you have tried hard to hide. You may feel shocked, or frightened even, that someone seems to know precisely what it is that you are seeking to deny or conceal.

Figure 4.13 shows some of the main factors present when you are working with others and how – if you tap these sources of information – their perceptions will enable you to revise your own.

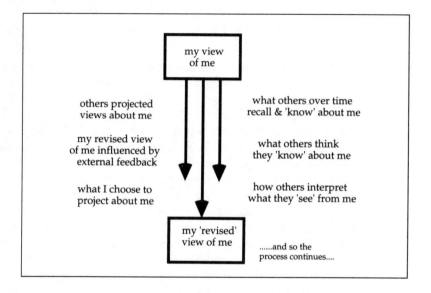

Fig. 4.13   Reviewing my sense of myself.

The key reason for having this chapter is my belief that the more you are able to appreciate, believe in and understand yourself the better it will be for you and for those in your care. Figure 4.13 shows a continuing process to revise the views of yourself through being more able, and prepared, to let in views from others. To reconsider, as it were, the internal dialogues, and rule books of before.

Use and build on the notes you have made so far. You will find them helpful in working through the remainder of the book and in your direct care work.

Each of us is doing the best we can, in our own particular way, and we don't get it right all the time. But the least we can offer others is our preparedness to engage with them as best we can, to give them our understanding for what they may be struggling with and trying to do. Your preparedness to respect, be generous to, and *be* with others are fundamental qualities in the building of constructive relationships. For a carer I would see these as prime qualities that will enable and facilitate the patient–carer relationship.

However your view of it all is only a part of the story. What now needs to be added onto the framework is first, you in relation to your age and stage in life and second how you relate and work with those around you. You in your life cycle will be discussed first and you and working with others will come in Part Three.

References

Beck, A. (1976) *Cognitive Therapy and the Emotional Disorders*, Penguin Books, Harmondsworth.

Brewin, C. and Antaki, C. (1987) An Analysis of Ordinary Explanations in Clinical Attribution Research. *Journal of Social and Clinical Psychology*, **5**, pp 79–98.

Ellis, A. (1973) *Humanistic Psychotherapy*, Julian Press, New York.

Kelly, J. (1955) *A Theory of Personality*, W.W. Norton and Co, New York.

Lane, D. (1989) *Attributions, Beliefs and Constructs in Counselling Psychology*, British Psychological Society, Leicester.

Meichenbaum, D. (1977) *Cognitive-Behaviour Modification*, Plenum Press, USA.

Further reading

Burnard, P. (1992) *Know Yourself*, Scutari Press, Harrow.

Burns, D. (1980) *Feeling Good: The New Mood Therapy*, Signet Books, New York.

Carson, R. (1983) *Taming your Gremlin* Harper & Row, New York.

Goffman, I. (1969) *The presentation of Self in Everyday Life*, Penguin Books.

Lane, D. (1990) *The Impossible Child*, Trentham Books, Stoke-on-Trent.

Luft, J. (1963) *Group Processes*, The National Press, Palo Alto.

Spinelli, E. (1989) *The Interpreted World*, Sage Publications, London.

Chapter 5
Life Stage Frameworks

Introduction

Our concerns, our ambitions and our preoccupations about life do not stay the same as we get older, they change. Sometimes we notice changes in our views or perspectives about things as they occur (for example, about having to be super-successful etc.) and we are able to adjust to them in a self-acknowledging way and with little apparent trauma. With other matters we may suddenly realize that a major life change has occurred, for which we were not prepared, such as middle age, or receiving senior citizen status. This shocks us into reappraising our life.

There will be some concerns that persist over time, such as needs for security, survival, affiliation and in being able to live as we wish to. It is also likely that we will have some need for a level of social contact that meets our preferences. Beyond these considerations different matters occupy our thoughts and perplex us as we get older.

For example, there are times when being accepted by others seems to push all else out of the way, and where the overriding question on our mind is 'what do I have to do to be accepted; to become part of the group, to be no longer different; to be not seen as an outsider?' At other times the concern that is uppermost may be about displaying tangible success, to be seen to have 'made it'. At yet another time the preoccupations are about the quality of our relationships with others; about *who* (not *what*) we are and about *how* we relate to ourselves and to others.

Our priorities and our preoccupations vary over time and influence our views about our value, our accomplishments and what we look for as satisfaction in life. Examples of these shifts of focus, and of personal meaning have been related, from various studies, to where we are in our life cycle.

We all go through a series of stages in our lives where what matters to us seems to change, depending on our age. The studies also suggest that moving from one phase of our life to the next is *not* a simple or straightforward progression. It involves giving things up with which we are familiar and on which we may have come to depend. It means coming to terms with new challenges and dilemmas some of which we may dread. It is also highly likely that in acknowledging our movement from one phase of our life to another we are forced to come to terms with the reality that we may not have achieved the position in life that earlier we had mapped out for ourselves. We may not have become the leader in the profession as we had predicted, or received the honours we had hoped for. Also, we may strongly resent losing our physical youth and appearance and adapting to this change is not always easy.

These ideas can help us to be clearer about what we see as important in our life now, as distinct from a few years ago. They are also very useful in helping you to understand a little more about some of the concerns and priorities your patients may have but have been unable to talk about.

Life stage models

The last 20 years have seen an upsurge of popular interest in the issues individuals face as they get older. This may have been stimulated by more interest in the quality of life and by the concerns expressed about the need to curb the excesses of society if the world is not to be irredeemably spoilt for future generations.

Theorists and writers have suggested that there are a number of distinct stages or phases that we go through and that these often have attendant personal crises or dilemmas which have to be confronted. An awareness of these life crises, and an understanding of the core dilemmas to be anticipated during different stages of a person's life, can throw more light on current patient issues. They can give you a contextual framework through which you can consider their needs more fully – as well as your own.

If, as Erikson (1985) suggests, '. . . every period of life has its own point, its own purpose. To find it and accept it is one of the most vital problems relating to life', then looking at life as a series of progressive phases of psycho-social development offers us a framework to look at where we are and what might be on our minds. This may help to explain why, for example, different age groups become preoccupied with quite different interests, worries and concerns.

There will of course be a whole variety of reasons why each of us sees things differently. The notion of these being in some way linked to our own life stage is an interesting and useful possibility. It is a further aid to understanding yourself better (and patients, colleagues, family and friends too).

Life stage models draw attention to:

- the likely phases of development during a person's lifetime,
- the predominant psychological pressures and dilemmas that are likely to characterize each stage,

- the possible personal issues and crises that need to be negotiated successfully for the person to adapt and move on to their next life stage.

While there will be individual differences in when, and for how long, we remain in each stage there appears broad agreement among those in this field that issues of profound psychological importance do arise for each of us at broadly the same times in our lives. We have to address and come to terms with them in some way.

You may have matters on your mind now that you are wrestling with which just seemed to come out of the blue. There may be a sense that you should be doing more, or that you need more independence, or maybe a sense that you have 'outstanding work to do' but you don't know what it is, etc. Without taking away your individuality look to see if your concerns are in any way similar to the concerns predicted by the following frameworks of someone of your age and stage of social development.

These ideas give you another perspective on your patients (and colleagues) who, in addition to their clinical condition, may be working through some transition issues in their coming to terms with a life stage transition.

Some approaches to consider

'Passages: predictable crises of adult life' (Sheehy, 1976)

This book became a bestseller in 1976 and Sheehy suggests that there are six *life passages* through which we move in our life. These are described in Fig. 5.1.

Sheehy also describes how, during each of the six life passages, each of us goes through four subtle changes in how we view and experience things. These are:

- in how we think about ourselves internally in relation to others,
- the proportion of 'safeness' to 'danger' we feel in our lives,
- our perception of time – do we feel that time is running out or that we have an inexhaustible amount of it available,
- there will be some shift at the gut level in our sense of aliveness or stagnation.

Levinson – 'Seasons of a Man's Life'

During 1978 Levinson *et al.* published the results of a series of field work studies that had begun, several years earlier, as a study of mid-life but which were expanded and developed into a more general theory of adult development.

1. *Pulling up roots*: moving away from parental care.

2. *The Trying Twenties*: where issues about personal identity, the nature of truth, the future and who it will be with are the primary concerns.

3. *Catch-30*: in this *passage* there can be an impatience and a discontent with one's achievements during the twenties and a new vitality against pre-conceived restrictions and a narrowness of life experience as people approach the age of thirty arises. It is a time of review and change and one of re-examination of what has been achieved – there is a rebelliousness and a sense of wanting to do things 'before it is too late'.

4. *Rooting and Extending*: here life becomes less provisional and more rational and orderly as – in the early thirties – we begin to settle down and put down roots; possibly having worked through some of the internal angst of the previous passage.

5. *The Deadline Decade* (35–45): here – at the cross-roads of the mid-thirties – is where even as we are approaching our prime we begin to see there is a place where it finishes; time starts to squeeze; there is a loss of youth, a reduction of the physical powers we had always taken for granted, the fading value and purpose of the stereotyped roles by which we had thus far identified ourselves, and a spiritual dilemma of having no absolute answers – any or all of these shocks can give this passage the character of a major existential crisis.

6. *Renewal or Resignation*: here equilibrium is regained and with it a new stability achieved as we move into new understandings of where we are and what is available to us 'friends become more important than ever, but so does privacy'.

Fig. 5.1 Sheehy's life passages.

He presents life as a process or journey (from birth to death) in which many influences along the way shape the nature of that journey and he introduces the notion of *seasons* as periods or stages within a person's life cycle. Each life cycle is seen as comprising of a sequence of eras, each lasting roughly 25 years. These are partially overlapping so that as a new one is getting underway the previous one is being terminated. His era sequence is shown in Fig. 5.2.

The journey is neither simple nor continuous, it has a changing flow and he suggests there are qualitatively different 'seasons' of life, each of

childhood and adolescence	[ages 0 - 22]
early adulthood -	[ages 17 - 45]
middle adulthood -	[ages 40 -65]
late adulthood -	[ages 60 -]

and he draws attention to four transitions from

early childhood	[during ages 0 - 3]
early adulthood transition	[during ages 17 - 22]
a mid-life transition	[during ages 40 -45]
a late adult transition	[during ages 60 -65]

Fig. 5.2   Levinson's Seasons and Transitions.

which has its own distinct character. He also notes that there are seasons within a single day (daybreak, noon, dusk, the quiet of night) , each with its own atmospheric and psychological character. It is quite a sophisticated model, each dimension of which seems to almost have a life of its own within the bigger picture.

He focuses mainly on the years from the late teens to the early 40s and his work has been instrumental in drawing attention to the major life changes that occur in the middle of the average life span. They roughly correspond to the division in Jung's terms (Jung, 1931) between the first and the second half of life. As Levinson says:

> The move from one era to the next is neither simple nor brief, it requires a basic change in the fabric of one's life, and this takes more than a day, a month or even a year. The transition between eras consistently takes four or five years – not less than three and rarely more than six. This transition is the work of a developmental period that links the eras and provides some continuity between them.

It is likely that the term 'mid-life crisis' came from Levinson's interest in looking at the changes that affect us during that period of our lives.

Nicholson's Seven Ages – *does your age really matter?*

By comparison Nicholson (1980) reports on a study during 1979–80 in Colchester which explored the subjective importance of a person's age to them. He noted that 'As the months went by and as a picture gradually built up about what age means to ordinary people it became increasingly clear that we are by no means slaves to our age, as the theory of the adult human life-cycle would have us believe' and he observed a tendency in other writers on the human life cycle to emphasize the difficulties that face people at different ages and an underlying assumption that, generally speaking, things get worse as years go by. His studies do not support this contention.

His research suggests that few people think that 'the actual me' changes much over the years of adult life and found that 'in as much as they are aware of ageing at all, most people see it as a means of coming to terms with themselves. As we get older, we get better at this, and become increasingly confident of being able to deal with problems and other people'.

Nicholson's findings suggest that we are not particularly burdened by our age or necessarily made gloomy by the prospect of growing older; that the changes to us are not simply the result of the passage of time alone, but rather because of major life events some of which may occur because of age but some of which can occur at any time.

He points out that life stages and their accompanying age bands are somewhat arbitrarily defined and they may only be important for most people if they begin and end with a major life event. Otherwise they may have little significance if unrelated to such a major concern. He suggests that the life stage theories – such as those popularized in *Passages* – are seriously at fault because they seek to normalize and specify that each individual will experience major shifts and traumas principally as a result of their age, irrespective of their individuality and previous life history.

Nicholson also challenges the suggestion that anyone can accurately anticipate, prescribe and describe the issues that each of us will be confronted with during the same time periods in our life. He does acknowledge however there to be underlying patterns of social development and change through life. Also that there are issues and concerns that may occur with particular prominence or frequency during particular stages of our life.

He emphasizes the subjective, rather than the normative, aspects of individual development and ageing. Also the importance of the effects of major life events on each of us, not just our progression to the next age stage or phase in the predicted developmental sequence. In these respects he is close to adopting a rather existential position. This is where the core focus is centred on the client's uniquely experienced concerns about their being-in-the-world which requires them to explore the meaning and importance for themself of what they have experienced. So far as patient care is concerned you would need to find out what the experiences meant to each patient. So far as *you* are concerned, think on.

Erikson's life cycle

One of the major contributors to exploring how we develop in the social world is Erik Erikson (1985) who has developed a psycho-social model of a person's development in which there are eight stages. Each of these stages attributes considerable importance to the individual's handling of relations with others. It is a developmental framework in which progression from one stage to the next is intimately grounded in what has gone before. Unresolved issues are carried onward within each of us as we pass through each stage of our development, and they continue to affect how we see things and what we do.

The model set out in *The Life Cycle Completed* is worth looking at more fully. It presents an account of how an individual's development rests on their successful adaptation to issues and dilemmas posed during a series of developmental stages. Erikson's approach sees a person's development arising primarily through their ability to handle increasingly complex, and broadening, interpersonal social contacts. He considers that there are significant non-instinctual determinants of personality. In other words, *we* can significantly determine who and what we are. He emphasizes the importance of the social and environmental determinants on personality. He uses case studies of people living in different circumstances and cultures to illustrate how their development is bound up with the settings in which they live.

According to Erikson,

> ... the child passes through a sequence of developmental phases, each phase having its own specific crisis... How the child meets each crisis is determined to a great extent by the solutions that are proffered or permitted by the parents and other caretakers, who in turn are influenced by society's traditions and ideologies.

His framework is outlined in Fig. 5.3.

The model provides a schematic overview of individual development and an anticipation of psycho-social crises to be expected. It provides a means of thinking about your issues in relation to which stage of development you see yourself. It alerts you to the likely crises and concerns that could be on your mind now, and in the future.

This is a dynamic model of human development and it suggests that each of us will experience dramatic shifts in emphasis about who and what we are and that these will – building on from the previous chapter – cause us to wonder who and what we are. Erikson's model offers a framework for you to use to review your notes from Chapter 4 and see if further insights emerge about where you are and what is on your mind.

Jung's first and second half of life

For Jung, the life span is divided into two halves – that before 40 and that afterwards and he considers that

Stages	Psycho-social crisis	Basic Strength	Core - pathology
I Infancy	Basic Trust vs Basic Mistrust	Hope	Withdrawal
II Early Childhood	Autonomy vs Shame, Doubt	Will	Compulsion
III Play Age	Initiative vs Guilt	Purpose	Inhibition
IV School Age	Industry vs Inferiority	Competence	Inertia
V Adolescence	Identity vs Identity confusion	Fidelity	Repudiation
VI Young Adulthood	Intimacy vs Isolation	Love	Exclusivity
VII Adulthood	Generativity vs Stagnation	Care	Rejectivity
VIII Old Age	Integrity vs Despair	Wisdom	Disdain

Fig. 5.3 Erikson's psycho-social model of development.

... when an individual reaches the late 30s or early 40s a radical trans-valuation occurs. Youthful interests and pursuits lose their value and are replaced by new interests which are more cultural and less biological. The middle aged person becomes more introverted and less impulsive. Wisdom and sagacity take the place of physical and mental vigour. His values are sublimated in social, religious, civic, and philosophical symbols. He is transformed into a spiritual man.... This transition is the most decisive event in a person's life. It is also one of the most hazardous because if anything goes amiss during the transference of energy the personality may become permanently crippled. (Jung, 1931.)

These notions of a higher purpose, a drive towards an actualization of individual potential are prominent feature of Jung's view of man. This emphasis on higher level aims, aspirations and transformations have a strong spiritual base. They act as a reminder of your aspirations and the importance of focusing on your future potential and the quality of life.

There is a calm simplicity in the notion of the two halves of a person's life span. While the profound shift of emphasis may not be seen overtly for many people that does not mean, perhaps in many subtle ways, that the shift of emphasis that Jung suggests has not occurred.

Ages of a manager

This is an altogether different framework and is related to your career aspirations and how these alter over time. The stages of development outlined so far are also likely to be reflected in how we see ourselves progressing in our professional life. By way of illustrating this I have included some work done by Kiechel (1987) which relates the main concerns we may have as a manager according to our age.

The age bands are as set out in Fig. 5.4.

> *The 20s – Proving yourself worthy:* The priority here is to demonstrate that you have what it takes to do the job. Research on the careers of professionals also showed that a willingness to accept direction, and expected acquiescence, from senior colleagues was looked for which contrasts with (see Erikson's Life Cycle) the moves the young adult wants to help define themselves as an independent person – so there is a potential conflict here between what we want to achieve as a developing person with what is often looked for from us when in the early stages of our career.
>
> *The 30s – Making your mark:* By this time there is a pressure to demonstrate one's worth and ability through promotion and professional/managerial accomplishment. There is a sense that the clock is running and that unless I can get there (wherever the person's aspirations are leading them) by 40 I may not get there at all! This may mean first becoming a specialist or an expert in a chosen specialist field. The 30s can be characterised by an almost frantic, obsessive and competitive wish to succeed in ways that will be observable to others.

The 40s – Wrestling with limitations: Most people just don't make it to the top and the agenda during this phase – for the great majority – is about learning to live and come to terms with this, and other, limitations. This period is an especially important one where the 'mid-life crisis' of Levinson occurs and the move into Jung's second (and more qualitatively oriented) half of one's life takes place. Thoughts of mortality, of what for the future, of possible career changes and of re-shaping aspects of one's life often emerge here prompted by a realisation of personal limitation. Dropping out emotionally and intellectually is a danger.

The 50s & the early 60s – Avoiding insularity: The challenge now becomes either coming to terms with one's achievements and abilities and/or learning to use one's influence and standing wisely. Developing and encouraging others, prudent leadership of one's responsibilities, insightful and appropriate self management: these occupy the mind at this time. A danger though is an increasing propensity to move into oneself, towards an insularity from colleagues and in one's outside relationships. If this can be kept in balance there is a tremendous professional resource available in these experienced professionals.

Not overly concerned with competition, personal power or a need to display influence they are a tremendous resource that can be tapped to coach, support and develop others within the organisation and profession. Their wish is that their expertise, wisdom and experience be recognised and used – that in this way they will be able to continue to be a valued and valid contributor.

and beyond – Wise guidance & calm: By this time it is possible to have achieved a perspective on the profession or the organisation that allows you to offer insights that few others can make. You are able to provide wise counsel, to offer a calming influence that will allow those younger than you to pause, understand more fully what they are dealing with and then decide.

Fig. 5.4 Kiechel's ages of a manager.

Figure 5.5 shows this visually. You may like to see where your age sets you on this and if the overall comments about that age band reflect your current position.

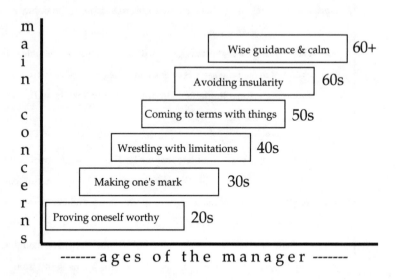

Fig. 5.5   The ages of a manager (Kiechel (1987)).

In addition to the descriptions in Fig. 5.5 our view on our career development will be influenced by a combination of the following:

(1)   where we are on our human life cycle (which phase, stage or season),
(2)   the particular experiences associated with our age group (for example remembering the assassination of President Kennedy, the BandAid concerts or the Thatcher–Reagan era),
(3)   the career life cycle (from training to more senior roles) which may or may not integrate with our human life cycle phases and pre-occupations,
(4)   major life events that we have experienced as 'landmark' events and that have then conditioned our subsequent life experiences (for example, childbirth and parenthood, death of a person close to us – especially if it was untimely or traumatic, significant personal successes, etc.).

This career progression sequence is best taken as an indication of how our preoccupations do alter. There will always be exceptions, over time as we wrestle with our achievements, our disappointments, our limitations and the contributions we feel we still have to make.

For many people what we do and how we progress at work is seen as a (perhaps *the*) principal purpose of our life. Therefore what happens at work, and in our professional life, holds immense personal significance for us psychologically. We can experience profound joy in work success and deep despair in disappointment that can seem to others out of all proportion to the event itself.

Using these ideas

Life stage models provide frameworks for considering your immediate concerns as part of your broader life context. Familiarity with these models may enable you to adopt a more holistic approach to your life and your current issues and preoccupations. With your patients the same applies and these models may help you to see and understand them with a sensitivity that you were unable to employ previously.

These perspectives acknowledge that individuals have changing and differing psychological and social preoccupations at different times throughout their lives. As we develop over time we seek to adapt to our new circumstances, conditions and realizations of who we are and what we are about.

These studies could lead us to conclude that we are rather passive parties in all of this; that we just slowly progress through a pre-determined life course with psychological obstacles and challenges to surmount. If we do well then we 'pass go' but if not we have to wait until we do surmount the obstacle and can then move on. I do not believe it is quite like this. Instead these frameworks offer a series of maps that can help us (and our patients and colleagues) to see and to make more sense of where we are and of the possible terrain ahead.

While there are differences between them there are a number of shared features that emerge:

- Life can be developmentally sequenced into a number of phases or stages.
- There are transition issues and traumas experienced in moving from one stage to the next.
- Each life stage has its own particular issues for the individual to address.
- Unresolved issues from earlier stages will impact on current and future stages and our ability to cope.
- Human life is essentially progressive, developmentally focused and forward looking.
- There is a continuing social-cultural dimension as an integral part of a person's life development.
- The progression is from simple to more complex maturation, learning and behaviour.

For your work with patients this material provides you with a number of frameworks that:

- can enable the patient's wider social context to be remembered and be taken more fully into account,
- can aid understanding of the importance of the patient's presented issues with regard to their age and possible life stage
- can provide ways of describing the processes of adaptation and change the patient may be experiencing,
- can alert the nurse to the possibility of future issues that may arise for the patient and with which they will have to contend.

References

Erikson, E. (1985) *The Life Cycle Completed* W.W. Norton and Co, New York.

Jung, C. (1931) *Collected Works: Vol 8, The Stages of Life* Princeton University Press, USA.

Kiechel, W. (1987) *Ages of a Manager. Fortune* 5 November 1987.

Levinson, D. *et al.* (1978) *The Seasons of a Man's Life*, Ballantine Books, New York.

Nicholson, J. (1980) *Seven Ages*, Fontana Paperbacks, Glasgow.

Sheehy, G. (1976) *Passages*, Bantam Books, Toronto, Canada.

Further reading

Bolles, R. (1981) *The Three Boxes of Life*, Ten Speed Press, Berkeley, USA.

Bridges, W. (1991) *Managing Transitions* Addison-Wesley, Reading, USA.

Lievegoed, B. (1979) *Phases: Crises and Development in the Individual*, Steiner Press, London.

Chapter 6
Working with Myself

By now you have amassed a lot of information about yourself, some of it surprising perhaps, some of it making you wonder about what else is waiting for you to make a note of. You may feel a bit excited or a little bemused and concerned.

If you notice that all of the notes you have made are positive then I would like you to think about that. It may be somewhat out of balance, and now might be the time to look again and make a note of some of the less positive attributes or feelings you carry around with you. Similarly, if you see that you have overwhelmingly recorded negative, or dismissive points about yourself please look again at your experience of yourself to see what strengths and positive features you have avoided. Don't give an unbalanced picture of yourself. See if there are now some additional positive attributes you have not recorded or overlooked.

This process of self review has not finished. It is the type of process that always continues. You now have quite a lot of 'leads' about yourself even though there is more work to come. For the moment the question is 'So what?' and 'How can I use it?'.

Question 1: So what?

If you have some understanding about what is important to you, and of what helps or hinders your ability to function in the world as you would wish, you have considerable knowledge at your disposal. If, on the other hand, you have very little understanding of how you behave and about what seems to help and hinder you in life then it will be more difficult for you to change. You may become frustrated or lethargic about things generally but not know why this might be or what is wrong.

I am not talking here about creating a world which is centred around you in a narcissistic way but where your self-knowledge and self-confidence can be exercised fully to shape and influence what is going on.

With a clearer view of yourself and what you do (such as including the positive and the negative conversations that go on as part of your internal dialogue) you will arrive at a more balanced and realistic picture of yourself. In turn this will help you keep in perspective the unexpected ebbs and flows of life and thus you may be able to tackle them with increasing confidence and resolve them when they arise.

The principal outcomes I see from this self-review are that you are more likely to:

- make more informed choices than before,
- have more of an idea of what matters to you,
- be more aware about what you are seeking out of life.

Much of this comes through the effort you have put in by being more open with yourself through:

- your increasing preparedness to listen openly to what you are doing (both in your actions and in your thoughts),
- watching and seeing more fully what is going on around you,
- making a commitment to look after yourself as a valued and valuable person.

These are essential prerequisites for you to care for and look after others. The logic here is that it is very difficult to care for others if you don't have a positive and realistic view of yourself. For this to be achieved you have to have looked at what you do, have some sense of what you are and be prepared to see the good and the bad, the strengths and the frailties, the rational as well as the irrational aspects of you as a person. In this way, not only can you reach a fuller awareness of yourself but you can also begin to appreciate more what life may mean for others (patients, colleagues and friends, for example) to be as they are.

Working as a nurse inherently provokes anxiety. Caring for those in physical and psychological distress such as patients, relatives and other carers, carries with it anxiety. The emotions of life and death are never very far away, nor are the big questions about life. There are questions about why me, why them, what is the purpose of it all, and what am I doing here anyway. Feelings of guilt perhaps, of great joy, humility and shame, to mention only a few, are always near the surface with you or with a relative or a patient.

There are two basic choices you can take in response to this. The first is to begin to acknowledge and then work with the emotionality of the nursing role. The second is to try and deflect or dismiss the emotionality of it all (perhaps as a way of coping with it).

This second option could be achieved by emphasizing the routines, the procedures, the tasks etc., that need attention thus taking away the focus from the patient. Another strategy for handling the emotional dimensions could be through confidently asserting that these dynamics are being handled and that 'it's all part of a day's work'. A somewhat stoic and perhaps heroic response which may or may not be accurate – but at least it can give an impression of coping.

If though, you respond by working *with* the emotionality inherent in the role, you have to consider what working with your patients emotionally means for you too. There will be questions about meaning, purpose, the unfairness the patients feel. Also the envy, jealousy and, at times, hostility that will be directed towards you because you will possess the things they want. For example good health, four limbs, a clear thinking mind, a position, social status and a profession.

By developing more of an understanding about yourself – as we have been exploring in this Part – can help you to confront and tackle some of the imponderable issues of life. But it will also help you to 'hold' and 'stay' with the issues and tensions generated by the patients in your care.

As a nurse you are continually confronting issues concerning the meaning of life and the 'spirit' of people in acute distress and adversity. These include the horror of some physical and psychological conditions, the failings and the strengths of people in distress and outcomes such as the 'good' patient dying and the 'difficult' one recovering.

Your personal challenge is to accept and work with a more aware view of yourself, and of your own issues, *and* be able to continue to undertake the nursing, caring responsibility of working with your patients as people rather than as cases of clinical conditions.

To be able to do this will enhance your nursing ability and you as you. But, many of the emotional protections built into the nursing role may need to be loosened, if not taken away, to allow the nurse as a person to come through, both for the benefit of their patients and for themselves.

Question 2: How can I use all this material about me anyway?

The first thing is to recall the sets of information you have built up about yourself, see Fig. 6.1. Some 'core' themes will run through this material.

- What I believe in   • What I like & don't like
- Some of my sensitivities • Some reflections on the past, current
- Where I am in life   & the future
- Some feedback about how others see me
- How I see the future   • How I think about & picture myself
- What I want to achieve • How I want to be
- Messages I give myself • Messages others give me

Fig. 6.1 Information about me.

There will be underlying messages about you that reflect and capture the essential aspects of you. If you had to make a note of these what would they mean for you? Look at the notes you have made so far, look at what you have read from the book. Now by focusing on yourself how would you sum up, capture, identify and describe yourself using the information you have now put together? What are the underlying descriptions that, taken together, reflect who and what you are? Make a note of the core descriptors as you see them in Fig. 6.2.

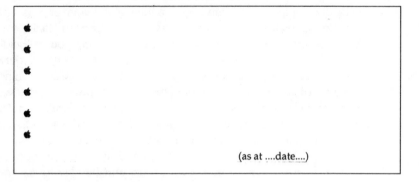

Fig. 6.2   My view of myself.

This is very difficult to do and it will probably take several tries. But it will be helpful because you can then begin to see yourself in a more complete way. This can throw more light on who you are and make more sense of some of the things you do, and those you shy away from given the opportunity.

What makes this activity different from previous times when you may have tried to describe yourself is that now you are drawing on the different sets of notes and reflections you have made. You need to look at those notes and see what they suggest about you. This is quite different to just pulling thoughts out of your head without any preparation.

If you don't like some of the messages you have set out in Fig. 6.2, look at them again. Assess if they are accurate and how, what and why you may want to start work on altering them. You may consider that each of these descriptors is a valuable aspect of you, even if you don't like all of them. Together they may present a complete picture of you as you know yourself even with the occasional wart! The messages in Fig. 6.2 can help to sketch a more rounded and realistic picture of you that you can then consider, explore and come to terms with.

A snapshot of me – now

I don't believe that we arrive in the world fully formed or that we don't have choices and opportunities open to us to alter events. I can see aspects of myself that have remained relatively constant over the years, although in earlier years I would have been unable to describe these with any precision. I can also see that I go about certain things differently now. I have learnt through experience ways that I now prefer to follow and that are relatively successful for me. Equally, I am clearer that I am not as capable as I might wish in other areas, that I still shy away from certain issues and find it difficult to address others.

I see myself as a mix of attributes, of skills and abilities, and that there remain areas that I recognize are not as I may prefer them to be. Nevertheless this is the way it is for me for the moment and I can still, in spite of imperfection, get along. At any point in time I work on the basis that I am where I am *but* that if I choose, I can alter some aspects about me if I really wish to. If I choose not to take action to change things I am telling myself that, for some reason or other, this is not the right time. However, if I have some insight into my own dilemmas and predicaments, then I do have the opportunity to work on aspects of me I want to alter when I am ready. Without this insight I don't have that choice. All I may realize is that I 'don't feel at ease', or 'something's wrong with me'.

Each time I reflect about myself I get different bits out and I put them together to build up a sense of me as me. I use these developing notions as working descriptions of me that help me to be clearer about who and what I see myself to be. I find it helpful and reassuring. I don't try to pigeon-hole myself or pretend that I can do everything, nor that I am perfect, merely the way I am. I have worries, am content in some ways yet not in others, but overall I have a sense of being more or less in balance with myself.

What sense do you have about yourself, and how do you feel about it all? May I invite you to do this for yourself now by pulling your thoughts together (see Fig. 6.3)?

You may want to use Fig. 6.3 as a basis on which to record those major aspects about yourself that have come through from your notes.

Pulling your thoughts and reflections together

You now have thoughts and ideas about what and how you do things; considerations about what you like or don't; thoughts about the type of relationships you like too. You will also have begun to notice what it is you do that helps or seems to hinder you in the building of relationships. You may also have found your thoughts returning to past experiences, or flashing forward to future possibilities, expectations along with fears and worries too.

These reflections – sometimes clear and vivid, at others times confusing, unclear and ambiguous – can often become clearer if they are linked together in a way that helps you to order them and to take a 'historical' overview of your life.

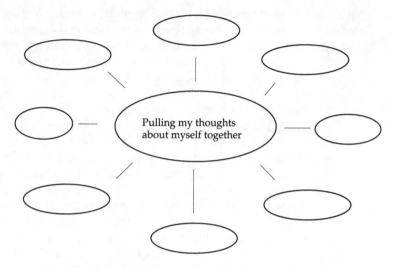

Fig. 6.3 Pulling my thoughts together.

To do this you need to make a note of the major events, episodes, feelings, difficulties, excitements, dramas and memories that come to mind when I ask you to 'make a note of your life'. So do this now, jot down the important things for you. These are things that happened and that you see as important.

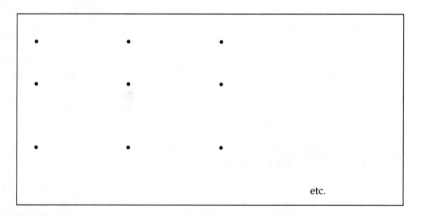

Fig. 6.4 Notes of my life: important and critical events, etc.

Your notes in Fig. 6.4 record major happenings for you that have resulted in you being who you are, and where you are today. These are stops, diversions and events along the way since you were born. You could look at life rather like a continuous journey with all its ups and downs, all its pleasures, surprises, disappointments and challenges and accomplishments.

Putting your views of yourself into a historical context puts critical incidents into a time sequence and you may notice (during at least some stages of your life) how some underlying patterns may have repeated themselves. I was amazed when I first did this some years ago to find there were some underlying patterns to a phase of my life of which I had not previously been aware. Once I had made those connections a number of other things fell into place. I was able to achieve a more balanced view about that time in my past.

Can you now make a start in doing this for yourself? Draw a straight horizontal line; the left end is when you were born and the right end is when you will die. Now look at the notes you jotted down in Fig. 6.4 and start to order then in an historical sequence along the line you have just drawn. You are now building up a life history line that shows all those happenings that have particular relevance and meaning for you. As you are doing this additional thoughts will come flooding into your head. They may be things you had forgotten, or brushed aside, when you were making your notes a few moments ago. You can also add them in.

The next stage – apart from starting again and selecting a larger piece of paper to do your next draft on – is to indicate if the events you recorded were positive or negative. You can do this by positioning them above or below the line. You can also think about the future too. What will be the major events you anticipate and will they be positive or negative in some way?

Figure 6.5 shows one example of a life line; the vertical line shows where the person is now.

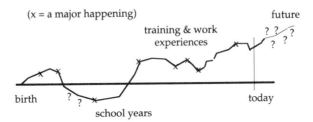

Fig. 6.5 Example of a life line.

In the figure I have shown how there were many ups and downs and several specific events that were very important in shaping my development to the present time. These are shown by the x marks in the figure. These can be anything that you see as important to you. I have listed in Fig. 6.6 some examples, not necessarily from my life, to prompt your own thoughts.

These are just some thoughts – the key is that you identify precisely those things that really mattered to you and which you feel have led you to become who you are now.

Positive Points	Negative Points
going to the big school	failing 11+
first bike	best friend left
first love	parents parted
accepted for training	the car crash
state registration	my first death on ward
coping with the emergency	depressive episode
etc etc	

Fig. 6.6 Examples of important life events.

When you feel it would be helpful you may wish to build up your own lifeline. Do it as fully and as honestly as you can. In that way you will probably notice some things about your own history that are new and some that are unexpected. When I first did this I was very surprised to see that in my teenage years there was a recurring pattern of not doing very well academically, which was then followed by an unexpected recovery. The pattern would then repeat itself. I was able to alter this but it was only many years later that I was able to see the pattern that I had been following. If I had seen it sooner I might have been able to do something about it.

You can use your life line(s) to do the following:

- think about where you placed your emphasis,
- notice underlying patterns about yourself,
- to see what you view as high points,
- to see what the low points are/were,
- note what seemed (if anything) to trigger life shifts,
- note questions that now occur to you about yourself.

You can see and feel what it means to look at yourself in this way. What does it reveal and disclose, what are the hidden messages that jump out at you? Is it painful, is it a great joy to have this way of looking at yourself and reminding yourself of all the things that have happened?

You may find that you will want to update your life line every few years. You may be surprised at how different they become as you change your perspectives on your experiences over time. For this reason, to get better insight, it is a good idea to keep earlier versions safely tucked away. After you have finished working and dating them, keep them hidden to stop yourself being overly influenced by 'what I did last time'.

Explaining your life line to someone else can be a very fruitful, and at times difficult, undertaking. They can help you to explain what has happened over the years and what the main messages are that you have taken away from this work. You may wish to think about this when you decide the time is appropriate.

In turn, you may find that a colleague will ask if they can show you their life line. How would you handle that? What would you say about their life line if they asked you? You may like to think about that now and consider what questions you would ask. The following are some examples to begin with:

- What is the overall message your life line gives you?
- Why do you think that 'X' was so important to you?
- What was it about the time 'Y' that was so . . . for you?
- Could you explain . . . a little more?

Do this with care, because they are sharing a great deal with you that is precious.

Concluding comments

This chapter has introduced some ideas about yourself that build on those you already have. As you go through the book you might like to return to these notes and update them accordingly. This will take account of more additional subtleties about yourself that you may have overlooked. Then you can use these thoughts to keep in mind your developing sense of yourself as you go forward.

Of course we don't exist and work in isolation. In many ways we define ourselves primarily in relation to others. Thus we move now – in Part Three – to focus on working with others and the problems, difficulties, joys and dilemmas that these raise for each of us.

Further reading

Pedler, M., Burgoyne, J. and Boydell, T. (1986) *A Manager's Guide to Self-development*, 2nd edn, McGraw-Hill Book Co, London.

PART THREE:
INTERACTIONS, INFLUENCE AND INTERFERENCE

In this part the focus moves from yourself to you in relation to others. Chapter 7 looks at some of the different types of relationships and expectations that centre around being a nurse and the expectations others can have of you in such an influential position. It offers some frameworks you may want to use to help you rethink and then to restructure your relationships and ways of working.

Working with others means having to decide what you want and then expressing your views so that others listen and then act on your guidance, wishes, or instructions. This is not always easy to accomplish. Either you may not make it clear enough to others what you want or perhaps the way in which you convey it is not strong enough for them to follow your lead. At the same time the other person will have their own wants and needs, and these will not necessarily coincide with yours. In these cases you will need to resolve differences to reach a viable outcome. These matters are considered in Chapter 8.

Chapters 9 and 10 focus on you in teams, groups and meetings and offers a number of practical perspectives for you to use. The differences between *leadership* and *management* are explored in Chapter 11. These are often rolled together when people talk about work behaviour, yet they are quite different.

Chapter 7
Relationships and Expectations

No matter how positive we feel about ourselves, or how confident we are in our ability to be successful, we live in relation to, and are partially dependent upon, other people around us. We are, as some would say, *social animals*. We cannot totally isolate ourselves from the effect of others on us or neglect the impact that our behaviour has on them. Much of our own sense of self, and relevance as a person, comes from the comparisons we make with others.

We put a great deal of effort and energy (both psychological and physical) into deciding how we want to appear to others, and in cultivating the impressions we want to create and sustain. In turn we notice, in great detail, the behaviours and adornments of those around us, which we then – consciously or unconsciously – compare and contrast with our own.

In our chosen vocation, our speech and in our declared aspirations we define ourselves through our similarity with and affinity to, or difference and disagreement from, others. We are relational beings and we are destined to act out our lives with, and around, other people. How we go about this affects the course and the quality of our life. It is therefore critical to know what we want from our associations with others and to have some idea of what type of relationships are there for us. To make our choices we need to understand and value ourselves. This is the understanding that emerged from Part Two.

There are two sections to this chapter – the first part (A) considers some aspects of the relationships and expectations between patients and their carers, and the second part (B) considers some of the anxieties and stresses experienced in caring for others.

A: PATIENT–CARER RELATIONSHIPS AND EXPECTATIONS

At the crossroads of care provision

In terms of contacts and interactions the position of a nurse is similar to that of a person strategically located on one of the main crossroads on one of the old silk and spice routes. These were the main routeways of the civilized world at that time, the great land transport and trading routes where precious cargoes were transported and business deals agreed, and also where powerful relationships were formed. All the time the watcher at the crossroads saw the people as they came and went with their many different loads, stories, customs, concerns, considerations, worries and needs. Many failed to notice the watcher sufficiently and perhaps took him for granted, yet he was an important part of the scene and helped it all run smoothly. The watcher as the carer is the helper, listener and soother as well as one qualified to give professional counsel and advice to the travellers and merchants of the trade routes.

In some ways I see the nurse in a similar position, at the main crossroads of the life routes of their patients. This may seem a bit fanciful and dramatic perhaps but it captures some important relational aspects of the nursing role that can be overlooked.

What would your version be of such a crossroads for a nurse or carer? Figure 7.1 offers a start.

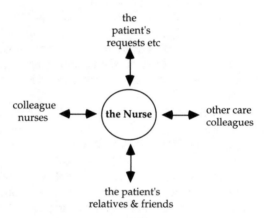

Fig. 7.1   At the crossroads of care provision.

This places the nurse in a central, crossover position. From here the nurse can take account and influence the priorities that are followed and the decisions and actions that take place regarding patient well-being.

While the silk route imagery may not be a perfect analogy, the nurse is there watching and providing a consistent and a coherent caring approach. This is not matched by any other professional in terms of the continuity of contact provided. Each day it is the nurse that sees the different needs of each patient ebb and flow throughout the day. The nurse is at the heart of it all the time. She is involved with all the comings and goings and with a responsibility of helping things happen, and of picking up and reassuring others along the way.

The key point is that much of direct care provision revolves around the nurse. She is influential both in guiding and in directing the pace and tone of the care environment. At the same time however, the nurse is also subject to tiredness and being worn out by the continual calls on her services and energy. In trying to meet the needs, wants and expectations of others, there is a danger of burnout and, psychologically, of the nurse losing herself and of neglecting her own needs.

To cope with this the nurse needs frameworks to:

- remind herself of what she is at the centre of,
- be more aware of the wide array of pressures, expectations and demands being made upon her,
- organize her conversations with patients,
- make explicit the different types of nurse–other relationships that arise during the course of her work,
- describe patterns of individual reactions to stress and trauma.

Without these aids it is possible the nurse will lose control of the situation and either go under, 'go into neutral' and cope in this way, or possibly leave the profession. None of these options benefits the nurse or the patient. The next section of this chapter suggests a series of frameworks and ideas that can help you to retain an overall perspective of what is being expected of you and of the changing nature of the nurse–carer relationship.

Purposeful relationships: the notion of contacts and conversations

One simple way of increasing your impact in working with others is to make sure you are clear about the purpose of that working relationship as soon as you can. Although you may initially think this is unnecessary, remember that when people work together there are usually several different purposes being played out at the same time. Unless these are clarified, confusion and relationship problems can be generated. Clarifying what you and others are there to do can help reduce confusion and competition, enhance effectiveness and reduce some of the strain on you at the centre of things.

Sometimes you may want to analyse what the purpose(s) is in your head. You can ask yourself 'what we are here to do'. At other times it will be necessary to either ask explicitly for clarity or state your understanding of what you are there to do and then see what that reaction elicits.

If you don't get into the habit of doing this you are at risk of:

- achieving far less than you otherwise could,
- being drawn into inappropriate uses of your time,

- role confusion (for you and possibly others),
- losing an opportunity to challenge what is being suggested (that is if you thought it inappropriate, etc.),
- losing your own sense of priorities,
- becoming frustrated when what you expected doesn't happen,
- reducing the likelihood of mutual collaboration.

One way of thinking about a professional relationship is to see it as offering scope for a whole array of *conversations* each for a different purpose. When you start to think in this way you have a framework you can use to make more explicit what you are trying to do. This clarifying of purpose can be done sensitively and positively and will act as a relief, especially so for anxious patients, because it is a simple and straightforward structure around which to frame their discussions with you.

Figure 7.2 shows what I mean and you can build it up in whatever way is most practical for you to use. You will see that I've left a few blank spaces for you to add in additional purposes for why people get together at work.

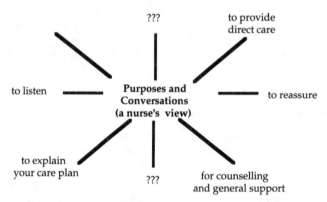

Fig. 7.2   Purposes and conversations.

I have drawn Fig. 7.2 from the perspective of the nurse working with a patient. The additional purposes you have for engaging with your patient need to be added onto this figure. Figure 7.3 is drawn from the patient's perspective and gives you some clues about the purposes the patient may have for engaging with you. You may want to compare and contrast the two figures. To what extent are there common purposes, and where are the differences since these are where tensions and conflicts may arise?

Being clear about the purpose of the working relationship suggests the types of conversations that are fitting and needed to fulfil the purposes identified. You have here a way of helping you to build up an

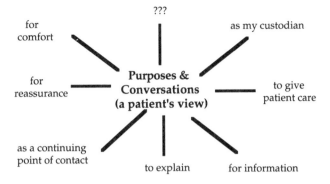

Fig. 7.3 Purposes and conversations: a patient's view.

appropriate patient–carer relationship and thereby guard against inappropriate and unreasonable expectations from both sides. You can do this by saying in a clear and apt manner what you are there to do and consequently define the types of conversations that are appropriate.

Build up your own version of this framework to make it work for yourself in your practice. You can then use it as an underlying framework to guide some of your work with patients. It can give them a clearer framework around which to structure the needs they have, the questions they want to ask and in clarifying their relationship with you as professional.

Elements of ethical conversations

Conversations between patients and carers are fraught with problems. The risk of mutual misunderstanding is heightened because of the complexity of the material being communicated, the anxiety for both you and the patient and the importance for the patient of what you are both telling each other.

What would you see as the factors inhibiting effective communication when a new patient and a carer communicate? You may like to use the format in Fig. 7.4 to jot down your view from both your own position and from that of a patient.

There are a great many barriers, confusions and impediments, not necessarily intended, that can get in the way and make it difficult for the nurse and for the patient to communicate freely.

As there are a lot of factors interfering with effective patient–carer communication, it is desirable to look for ways and means of reducing miscommunications and misperceptions. There is also a need to increase the chance of more accurate communication. One very useful approach has been developed by Eric Shepherd (1994) who uses the mnemonic RESPONSE as a way of highlighting key components of from the **patient's experience**   from the **nurse carer's perspective**

- •   - •

- •   - •

- •   - •

- •   - •

- •   - •

Fig. 7.4   Inhibitions to effective patient:carer communications.

respectful and responsible carer–patient communication. The components are shown in Fig. 7.5.

Each of the words refers to an important quality of your communication's tone, style and focus with patients. The features identified are easy and ethical in their intent. Together they provide a way of remembering what to offer your patient when you are working with them.

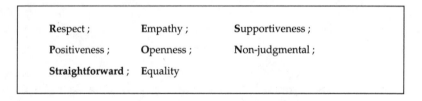

Respect ;	Empathy ;	Supportiveness ;
Positiveness ;	Openness ;	Non-judgmental ;
Straightforward ;	Equality	

Fig. 7.5   The RESPONSE framework for ethical conversations.

This framework has been developed from teaching medical students and you may find it helpful to use this framework to guide your own thoughts, reflections and conversations with patients, colleagues and friends. This gives you another means of self-monitoring your client contacts. You can also use the framework to prepare for forthcoming discussions with patients etc and also use it to run through beforehand what you plan to say and then see if your ideas meet the RESPONSE criteria.

In addition to following these eight critical attributes of effective, direct face-to-face communications, remember that *how* you relate to someone has a massive influence on their understanding of what you are saying. For example, you can talk about being respectful and about being non-judgemental but the way in which you are actually treating the other person could demonstrate quite the opposite. If this happens others will believe what they *see* you do rather than what you *say*. The importance of congruence in communications is discussed in Chapter 8.

Perhaps the single most important and effective attribute you can display in building effective communications with others is *attentive listening*. This happens when you focus all your attention on trying to appreciate and then understand the other person's point of view. Often the words *active listening* are used to describe this attribute. I prefer *attentive* listening because it makes the placing of your attention onto the issues of the other person in an attentive way more explicit. Attentive listening remains a cornerstone for effective professional practice, see Chapter 8.

A model for conversation management

If you are busy in the clinic, on the ward, or on a visit, or in an out-patients department you may have found that trying to communicate in a quick, and perhaps incomplete way, because you are rushed, actually causes you to spend more time with patients than intended.

By trying to go that bit faster you may often find that you end up going more slowly. This is because the patient either doesn't understand what you are trying to do or say, or they may feel hurried and resist your pressurizing them. They may become more confused, frightened and possibly angry and unhelpful. This may mean you then have even more work to do to reclaim the situation, restabilize and calm the patient so that they become more receptive.

Far better to plan your intervention in advance and then take it at a speed that best meets the needs of the patient and your time available. Every time you meet your patient several distinct stages are involved in that engagement, each of which requires some attention. I have set out in Fig. 7.6 the sequence and I advocate a progression through each until your work is concluded. Some of the stages noted below require very little time – perhaps less than a minute. But if they are omitted they can cause confusion or unease in your patient which will interfere with the care you are seeking to provide.

This is a five-stage sequence from the starting up of the conversation/ treatment episode, etc., to leaving the patient in a settled state and their having understood and been involved in what has taken place. Figure 7.7 shows how it looks graphically. On the left of Fig. 7.7 I have shown how the role of the carer changes from initiating and (later) concluding the patient contact to one of collaboration *with* the patient during the middle stages of the process. The five stages are displayed in Fig. 7.6.

You can use this as a basis to underpin and organize your conversations with patients into a series of linked stages each of which builds on and from the previous one.

(i) A Contact Stage: when there is contact and formal engagement again with the patient – this will cover introductions when the initial contact is made – but needs to be covered each time the patient is attended to, then there is

(ii) Specifying Purpose Stage: a need to convey and confirm the specific purpose of that particular meeting allowing for – and responding to any – questions, queries, worries or doubts that may be raised, before moving onto the next stage which

(iii) Task Completion Stage: is about completing the task or procedure to be done, providing support, guidance and encouragement as needed, following this is a need to

(iv) to review and confirm that the specified purpose has been satisfactorily completed and to monitor this: the patient may need some attention and care to re-stabilise them once again before the nurse moves away before

(v) the nurse formally confirms completion of the care programme or task etc. before finally leaving the patient in an acceptable state

Fig. 7.6   Five stages of patient contact.

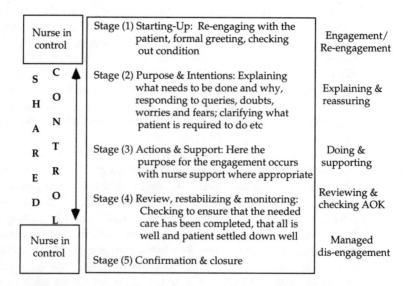

Fig. 7.7   A five-stage model for patient contact.

Stages (1) and (2) can get neglected, or very tersely attended to. This can result in that treatment starting even though the patient may be unclear what is going on, why you have come to talk to them or what precisely you want them to do. They may feel they are being discouraged from asking the questions they really want to pose. They may be unfamiliar with some or all of the carers on duty. This may lead them to feel as if they have no life of their own, that they are there merely to be treated like an object. In short, that they don't seem to matter.

Although the diagram is about carer–patient contact it can also be applied to relationships between professional colleagues. It takes little time to acknowledge a colleague, to explain today's priorities and allow an opportunity for them to engage and to become a part of the interaction and not just be a passive recipient of information. I don't know to what extent the needs of the nurse, or other care professionals are, in these respects, sufficiently acknowledged and met. My assumption is that a lot remains to be done to encourage and reward better relationships at work.

Realistic and unrealistic expectations

In addition to simplifying your conversations and clarifying their purpose, you need to be aware that patients and colleagues will have a host of expectations about you and the work you do. Some of these are reasonable, achievable and quite realistic but there are also likely to be some which are not. Yet they will, nevertheless, be held by some of those with whom you work.

From my experience too little attention is given to thinking about the different types of relationships looked for and the wide range of expectations that are held by others for their nurses. I think this leads to confusion, neglects issues of major significance and probably generates considerable stress. Some of this could be avoided when nurses strive to meet the unrealistic expectations placed on them by others, sometimes by themselves. Let us then think about expectations and different models of nurse–other relationships.

As you are so central to the care of patients it should not come as a surprise to be reminded that you occupy a special role in the life of a patient or client. They need not be your clients or patients either for the expectations they hold about nurses, in general, to be put onto you. In the mind of many patients you are quite special. You occupy a privileged role (i.e. looking after them, and they expect you to know what needs to be done and how to care for them, even if they don't know you, or you them. In their stress and dependency they will look to you and expect that whatever they need to be made well again will be forthcoming.

Perhaps I am overstating the case but in general terms I do not believe I am too wide of the mark. If patients see you as so critical to their care, their survival even, they are likely to expect a great deal from you. It is to your advantage, and well-being, to be prepared for the sort of expectations they have of you.

What follows is a simple method you can use to identify some of the expectations patients (and others) have. These will also influence the demands they will make on you, their perceptions of what you are doing and their experience of the nursing care being provided.

The first step is to put yourself in the patient's place. You can decide if this is to be an in-patient or an out-patient. Now jot down what you think they expect from you as their nurse. Be as frank as you can. Put down all that comes into your mind even if it seems a bit far fetched or silly. What you are trying to do is to get an idea of what might influence their relationship with you. You may like to use the format in Fig. 7.8 as a way of showing the different expectations you noted.

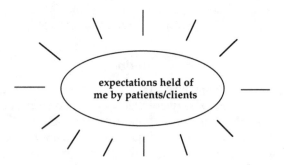

Fig. 7.8   Patient expectations of nurses.

In Fig. 7.9 I have shown some of the expectations that came into my mind and it is quite surprising how much can be expected of you in your role. It may not seem realistic to you, but from a patient's point of view such expectations become very real.

Not every patient will view you in the same way. But if you added all of their expectations, wishes, wants, fantasies and confusions together I am sure the expectations that I show on Fig. 7.9 are only a few of those held by patients.

You may be surprised at the range of expectations shown. Some of them may seem rather far-fetched, yet in my work with managers, nurses and other professionals these are the sort of comments that have arisen for discussion. You may want to see how close mine are to the expectations you noted on your diagram too. You might want to combine the two diagrams into one that reflects your experience of patients' expectations.

The key point is that the expectations which patients, and colleagues, hold dramatically affect the relationship you will have with them. They will base their assessment of you on the expectations and assumptions they hold. Therefore, unless you can clarify what they are expecting,

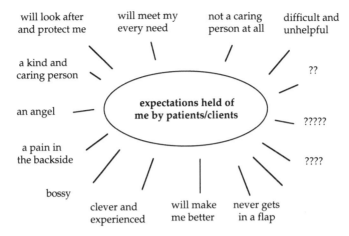

will look after
and protect me

will meet my
every need

not a caring
person at all

difficult and
unhelpful

a kind and
caring person

??

an angel

expectations held of
me by patients/clients

?????

a pain in
the backside

????

bossy

clever and
experienced

will make
me better

never gets
in a flap

Fig. 7.9 Possible expectations of nurses by patients.

and help them to redefine unrealistic or inappropriate aspirations into realistic ones, they are unlikely to see you as a valid or competent professional. They will judge you on their terms of what they want and not on what you can reasonably deliver.

If you are to tend even more carefully to the needs of your patients – and to your own needs – you will need to elicit the full range of expectations that are likely from patients. Through doing this you then create opportunities to reshape what is and is not appropriate and relevant. You will be able to guide your patients accordingly, and reinforce to yourself what you are there to do.

The next step is to think about your own expectations of being a nurse and providing care for and with others. Note down as many of your thoughts as you can. Make a list of what it is that being a nurse means to you. Be as frank and straightforward as you can. You are trying to make as explicit as possible the image that you take around with you in your work. Your notes can include different types of roles, different types of caring attributes, as well as some of the fears and worries that are part of your role.

Give yourself some time to do this because there may be a few surprises that pop up and also some thoughts that you would prefer to hold back. I would encourage you to note what these are as well, because they may help you define your ideas and feelings and put them more explicitly into place.

You don't have to record all your thoughts onto paper, but make a note of what comes to mind. They can help you to put things that were confusing or remain unresolved into a clearer perspective. You may like to transfer your thoughts onto the diagram displayed in Fig. 7.10. This type of figure can make it easier to see similarities and differences in your thoughts.

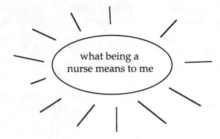

Fig. 7.10 What being a nurse means to me.

You now need to look more closely at what you recorded in Figs 7.8 and 7.10 to see if they make sense to you and if they are realistic given all you know. Look initially to see what each looks and feels like. What would you now want to add in; what would you want to alter? Would it simplify things if you re-ordered some of the individual items and clustered similar ones together? Are they compatible or are they mutually exclusive? If so what difficulties does that raise for you as a nurse?

So, re-work your notes and thoughts to make the most out of them that you can. One way is to compare side by side the expectations diagrams and make a note of how you feel about them. For example, does it come as a shock to see written down some of the unreasonable expectations that patients have of you as a nurse, or have you been fully aware of these all along?

See which expectations seem reasonable and *realistic* for patients to expect from you. Also which expectations do you consider are realistic for you as a nurse. Having done this, see if any of the expectations you have listed seem *unrealistic* in any way. This may be because you as a nurse cannot possibly fulfil the expectation stated or there may be some attributes or qualities that are not possible to have to the extent expected, or the patient may be expecting the impossible.

Having completed this you are now in a position to rewrite your initial lists into the summary in Fig. 7.11.

When you look at the unrealistic expectations/thoughts list, ask yourself where those items might have come from. If you do have an idea about their origin it will also give you a clue about how to dispel them. For example, a patient may have some unrealistic expectations which have come from the media or films. You can therefore, in an appropriate way, begin to explain what actually happens in practice and what you can and cannot do.

You may have noted down some unrealistic expectations that you have for yourself as a nurse. These may have come from what others have told you during training etc. They may be views about yourself (e.g. I must be perfect; I'm not good enough: You have to be strong, etc.) that

	Patients' View of me	My View of me	
(a) reasonable & realistic expectations	•	•	
	•	•	
	•	•	etc.
(b) unreasonable expectations.	•	•	
	•	•	
	•	•	
	•	•	etc.

Fig. 7.11 Summary of expectations.

have come from other times. Again by identifying them it becomes possible for you to re-examine their validity as you see them now. You can start to think about how to reduce their unhelpful or restricting influence. You may want to refer back to some of the material you covered in Part Two.

Also, when you look at the unrealistic list what effect does that have on you? How do you feel about the possibility of patients having such expectations? Whatever you have jotted down it is very likely that some of the items are just not feasible; or that you would have to be a superperson to achieve them. Now if you didn't have any idea about the possibility of patients having such unrealistic perceptions of what you are there to do you may have found that you rarely met the needs of some of your patients, whatever you did. But that you were unable to figure out why!

The consequences of all this are significant in that:

- your lists and diagrams can help you to appreciate what the patient may be concerned about and be expecting from you,
- if you have a clearer sense of what being a nurse means for you you can then use this to guide you in your work; start to reject contrary notions etc. and be more assured in your practice and in yourself.

This is another way for you to reduce some of the pressure you may feel under. At the same time it will give you an opportunity to re-assess some of your own expectations and those that colleagues may hold about you. At some stage you may find it helpful to share some of your notes, thoughts and ideas with colleagues and use it as a type of stress relief device.

Fundamental needs from our relationships with others

Some of the expectations you have been noting could be related to some of the fundamental needs Argyle suggests we look for from others (Argyle, 1967). He has identified eight needs which people attempt to fulfil in their relations with others, as shown in Fig. 7.12.

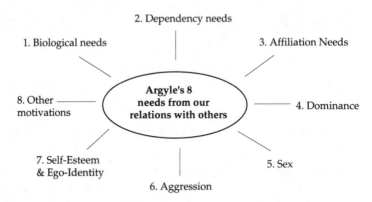

Fig. 7.12   Argyle's relationship needs.

He suggests that these needs underlay much of what goes on between people. You may want to see to what extent Argyle's eight needs are reflected in Figs 7.8 and 7.11 and underlay the expectations you noted. For example, are there any of Argyle's needs that feature more prominently than others for patients? If this is the case it may be helpful to keep Argyle's ideas in mind when working with patients and for you to be aware that their expectations, and reactions, could reflect underlying needs such as those proposed by Argyle. Are there any of Argyle's needs that don't feature on your lists and, if so, why might this be? From his list the need for sex is the one that is not appropriate for nurse–patient relationships. Yet it does not mean it will not feature, or covertly underpin the interactions that occur on the surface. Look to see how his eight relationship needs relate to your reflections.

You may also like to think about the most important people close to you, from any part of your life. You can then see what you need and what you actually receive from them using Argyle's eight needs as a guide. In certain cases you may be able to secure precisely what you are looking for; with others there may an imbalance or a gap. You may be able to identify that there is something lacking in the relationship, or that there is an imbalance.

If you are clearer about how things are going you can begin to consider why that may be. Then you can decide what, if anything, you may be able to do to change or rebalance the situation (see Fig. 7.13).

the relationship	the core need I want met	Is/isn't being met	Possible reasons why	Options to rectify

Fig. 7.13 Balancing the relationship

Now look at the relationship from the perspective of the other person. What do you think they are looking for or expecting from their relationship with you? Are their expectations realistic, appropriate and reasonable? Is there a shared need you both want from the relationship?

This approach can highlight a needs-mismatch very quickly and alert you to re-educate, re-examine or explore the expressed (or underlying needs) more fully.

Finally, you can use this model to

- reflect on who is important to you but with whom you haven't yet established an appropriate relationship,
- identify people you may have omitted altogether but who nevertheless are important to you,
- look at the overall pattern of needs and wants that are important to you at this time.

So, what are you there to do?

Given the differing expectations you have already noted it may be relevant to reconfirm what it is you are there, as a nurse, to do for the overall care of the patient. Is it to do a series of specific tasks, to keep the patient safe, to give emotional support; or perhaps to follow instructions, keep the doctors happy, avoid mess, keep things quiet and tidy or ... what?

One way of looking at your role would be to view it as spanning a care continuum which at one end involves delivering the determined treatment plan whereas at the other end it is about providing a totally integrated full care rôle to a patient. Figure 7.14 shows what I mean.

This continuum suggests a series of specific rôles you need to be able to cover depending on the circumstances of each patient. Your aim would be to work across the full range of this continuum.

By way of contrast, summarized below are two very different models of nursing care that can be followed:

(1) to look after – keep secure – control – containment – directive care – patient as object – emphasis on completion of allocated nursing tasks – power rests primarily with the nurse; and/or

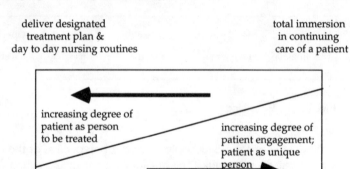

deliver designated
treatment plan &
day to day nursing routines

total immersion
in continuing
care of a patient

increasing degree of
patient as person
to be treated

increasing degree of
patient engagement;
patient as unique
person

Fig. 7.14 A care continuum.

(2) to look after – keep secure – monitor and review – engage and involve patient – directive and collaborative care decisions – emphasis on patient as person – emphasis on completion of nursing tasks with overriding emphasis on patients' needs – more equal power between nurse and patient.

These two different schema have implications for what it would be like to be the patient and to be a nurse under such care regimes. In the extreme, they can represent very different philosophies for providing health care. I may have contrasted them too sharply and there will be models of care that combine components of both of these. But remember how very different the experience of being a nurse and of being a patient will be depending on the tone, the ward or clinic culture, and the philosophical model of care that is being followed.

One way of explaining to patients the different roles you have to cover as a nurse is to look for a way of clustering them that makes sense to patients and their relatives. One such model is shown in Fig. 7.15. You could use this as a basis from which to develop your own way of discussing the different things you do.

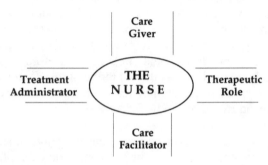

Care
Giver

Treatment
Administrator

**THE
NURSE**

Therapeutic
Role

Care
Facilitator

Fig. 7.15 Four role clusters.

The figure shows four core responsibilities that fall to nurses to deliver. The balance of attention varies between them depending on the type of nursing involved, the seniority of the nurse and the health setting concerned. While there is some overlap between some of these four roles I see them as follows:

(1) *Care giver:* Direct provision of bedside care, monitors and has responsibility for full nursing care of the patient.
(2) *Treatment administrator:* Completes treatments primarily as determined by others, emphasis on care tasks rather than whole patient orientation.
(3) *Care facilitator:* Works with the patient to facilitate recovery, adjustment to their condition etc.
(4) *Therapeutic role:* Functions in a more engaged therapeutic role (while still in general hospital) with patient rather than task focused nursing care.

If you think back to your current work, what is the approximate proportion of time you spend in these roles? I realize other things take your time but if you had 100 points to distribute between these four how would you say your time was spent? Use Fig. 7.16 to record your distribution.

My current speciality	Care Giver	Treatment Administrator	Care Facilitator	Therapeutic Role
	...... points	...... points	...... points	...... points

Fig. 7.16 Where the time goes now.

If you were now to look at these activities from the point of view of their impact for the patient's longer term recovery and care, would there be any difference in where you would then choose to direct your attention? This will vary depending on the speciality concerned and the severity of the patient's condition, however, bearing these points in mind, how would you distribute your attention using the 100 points again in Fig. 7.17.

If there is a change of emphasis ask yourself why this is. Does this suggest current practice should/could be altered in the interest of longer term patient benefit? If, on the other hand, you see no change necessary, what other roles in addition to the four highlighted would it be constructive to look at in the same way?

My current speciality	Care Giver	Treatment Administrator	Care Facilitator	Therapeutic Role
	......points	......points	......points	......points

Fig. 7.17 Source of impact for longer term recovery/care.

There is a need to identify what a nurse does that makes the difference (over and above administering direct clinical care) to a patient's care. What is it that is really very special that a nurse can do, in ways that other equally skilled and professional carers do not, or cannot do, that helps recovery and builds up a patient's resilience and belief. It is likely that there *are* things that nurses can do (and be) that can have a profound effect on patient belief and recovery but which are not in themselves clinical.

B: ANXIETY AND STRESS IN CARING FOR OTHERS

Personal anxiety and nursing care

In addition to the technical and professional standards and skills of the nurse a great deal revolves around the rapport and the quality of the nurse–patient relationship. While there will be professional standards and agreed care practices in place to ensure that all patients are received appropriately, treated with respect and cared for in a professional manner, the qualitative aspects of care fluctuate and remain an elusive, but influential, dimension.

Sometimes this will be because the patient is so tense and fearful, or conversely so desperate for care, that this impedes or blocks the building of this extra quality of nursing care. At other times it can be from the nurse that the blocks and barriers are put in place. This can be due to the patient's condition, perhaps because of other issues that are unresolved or are diverting that nurse at that time. This is not to suggest that good clinically competent and appropriate nursing care will not be provided. However, it could mean that the additional qualitative component to that caring relationship will not be present as fully as it otherwise could be.

It may be *anxiety* that gets in the way of the qualitative relationship. There may be worries in the patient's mind about their condition or pending treatment. The nurse may worry about the patient and yet be determined not to show any anxiety. The anxiety of being vulnerable and mortal is something worth considering in more detail. While it affects all of us it is one of the topics often dismissed as morbid, or pushed aside to be discussed 'some other time'. However as a nurse you will through the nature of your vocation, continually be reminded of this yet probably look for ways of not being overwhelmed by it.

What are the triggers to anxiety in nursing? It would be helpful if you could make a note of what causes you anxiety at work. It helps to do this with a colleague, especially if you want to build a more authentic working relationship with them. It may bring to light unrealistic views you have about the work you do and possibly about each other. To your great surprise you may also discover that, while there will be differences between you and your colleagues, your concerns and anxieties are similar to theirs.

If you can make a note of some of the situations which cause you anxiety you may also be able to describe how this shows itself. It may be that you try not to show any anxiety to others, perhaps preferring to try to bottle it up. It may be that you do things to provoke a scene where you are then able to get it out of your system for the time being but in a disguised form. You may have a variety of strategies for coping with anxiety , or maybe you keep it to yourself and you just go quiet. It may be that you become very meek or possibly you take sick leave to retreat physically for a time in a bid to protect yourself.

Whatever you do, make a note for yourself. You can use your own honesty to look again at how you experience anxiety-provoking situations and how you deal with them. One thing is certain; whatever anyone says, we *all* get anxious (although to differing degrees) at times. At some stage we all have to address the issues of human frailty and mortality that you see and work with on a regular basis.

If you can be clearer about how you respond, you may get ideas and support about how to reduce the effects of such anxiety in the future. Figure 7.18 gives a format to work from.

If the work of the nurse carries with it inherent anxiety, a balance needs to be struck between becoming immobilized by the feelings and

Causes of anxiety	How it shows itself	How I protect myself
1.		
2.		
3.		
4. etc.		

Fig. 7.18 Sources and responses to anxiety.

the emotions encountered (within yourself and from others) or becoming blasé and 'cut-off' from these experiences as a way of handling them.

The cultivation of inner understandings, of personal strength and humility are important as you develop your professional clinical understanding and expertise. At the same time, maintaining your internal integrity and cohesion is also important.

It may seem to you that the nature of the nursing role is one that is 'cradled in anxiety', as Isobel Menzies (1970) noted many years ago and at times this may prove almost too much to bear. The choice you have will be either to work with that anxiety or try to deny it. Working with it means looking for ways that will help you to acknowledge and 'stick with it' and not try to pretend it is not present. The second possibility is to decide that the most productive move is not to address the anxiety you are feeling but to push it away for the time being. Both these options can be more constructive than trying to pretend all is fine. This is a denial and can cause problems in the future. Figure 7.19 contrasts these two choices, to work with it or deny its presence.

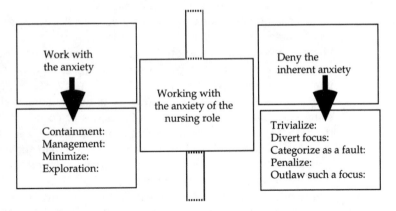

Fig. 7.19 Two responses to anxiety provoking situations.

Being in hospital – either as a patient or as a carer – is a cause of fear and anxiety. We don't always know what will happen to us, we don't always believe what people tell us about our condition, and we are reminded of our vulnerability. How we come to terms with this makes a considerable difference to our ability to cope with our own, and others', worries and concerns.

Just being in a hospital poses a threat to patients' self-esteem. They lose their independence and freedom of action, and are denied (temporarily at least, and for valid reasons) their daily routines and rituals. In place of these 'losses' the patients have foreign and unfamiliar routines and procedures, ones they may not want imposed upon them. All of this triggers fear and anxiety and in turn this can communicate itself to the nurse which in turn can trigger, or amplify, the nurse's own worries and anxieties.

In both the patient and the nurse, feelings of worthlessness, helplessness, fragility and vulnerability are likely to be induced. For the patient there may also be some feelings of guilt at being ill; of leaving others in the lurch together with fear of being dependent on strangers and of being unprotected.

Figure 7.20 shows some of the reasons why patients, and some staff too, begin to feel angry and sometimes become aggressive when in hospital. Given this scenario, how do you as a nurse help and support patients and their visitors? (Visitors may also show their anger, worry, fear, guilt and overall unease, and this could exacerbate the condition of an already anxious and vulnerable patient.)

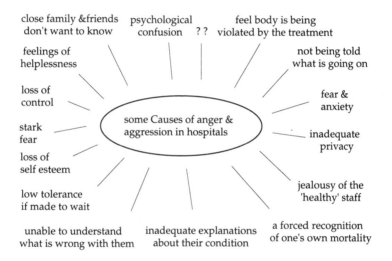

Fig. 7.20 Some causes of anger and aggression in hospitals.

One way is to be as clear as you can about your issues, strengths, worries and your belief in yourself as a caring professional and as a person. Building towards this is a sound way of acknowledging and working with the concerns of your patients and professionally supporting them without being pulled into their trauma.

Who I want the nurse to be

Patients build up powerful images of their nurse–carers whom they see along with their doctors as at the centre of their health care universe. In subtle ways they will communicate some of these images to their carers who (perhaps unknowingly) may begin to act them out.

Given the last section on the vulnerability of the patient and the patient–nurse susceptibility to anxiety, what images do you think the patient might have about their carers? Try to put yourself into the position of the patient. How might they come to see (and perhaps experience) you as their nurse?

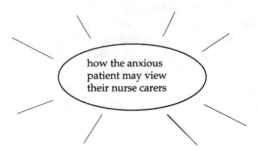

Fig. 7.21   How the anxious patient may view their nurse.

My list is as follows:

- as a guru
- as a problem solver
- as oppressor
- as domination
- as a guide
- as a magician
- as a saving angel
- as a wizard
- as life planner
- as true friend

- dependence
- as another person
- as a 'mate'
- as a cold professional
- as the high priestess
- as available for seduction
- as a confidante
- as a nurse professional
- as a protector
- as a counsellor

It is not unusual for the patient to develop strong relationships with, and images of, their carers. These are however of a very particular type and need to be managed by the nurse with great skill to maintain professional boundaries and limits. For example, the nurse will always be friendly but this does not mean she is a friend in the normal definition of that term. It should be recognized by the nurse that there is a significant power differential in favour of the nurse. This could leave the patient particularly vulnerable to suggestions in their dependent condition.

This can give rise to feelings of intense emotional attachment and regard for the nurse that can be difficult to cope with. This is especially so if the nurse is experiencing interpersonal difficulties with colleagues or others outside work. The vulnerability – and *captivity* – of the patient therefore places a high responsibility on carers being able to look after their patients with integrity and adhere to professional boundaries. In many ways the dependent patient–caring nurse is similar to the parent–child relationship.

It may, for example, be prudent professionally to work with the patient as if they were a dependent child. This is not in terms of their mental accomplishments and experience, but in terms of the physical care needed and their lack of awareness of the hospital and clinical world. However, the carer does not have the rights and privileges that a parent has with their child. The carer–patient relationship is altogether different even though it has similarities with dependency and vulnerability of the patient and need for physical care.

As the patient is in a dependent relationship so is the nurse vulnerable to their patients. The nurse is vulnerable to the inherent pressures of the job, to the many intimate tasks that are to be performed and to the calls on them made by patients, colleagues and others. The nurse is especially vulnerable to other professional colleagues more senior to them, and responsible – to some degree – for those less experienced.

Given these mutual vulnerabilities, what is interesting is the way in which the nurse can be a counsellor to the patient and how, in turn, the patient can be a counsellor to the nurse. Precisely because of the heightened sensitivity of the patient and the opportunity the patient has to observe, monitor, and review what is going on around them, they will pick up many clues about their carers.

Listening attentively to, and learning from, the patient is not only tapping a source of potential wisdom but therapeutic for the patient and the nurse alike. Just as the patient will resent their collective status as 'patient' so the nurse will resent their anonymity as 'nurse'. Both parties have a right and a need to be recognized as people by each other (and by colleagues). While working within the necessary professional boundaries, if the patient–carer can listen to each other, this process will help to ensure that the essential humanity and uniqueness of being in a hospital (both as patient and as carer) is not lost or denied.

Relating to relationships

Meeting your needs in any relationship is not a straightforward matter because of the number of influences actively affecting the course and the nature of that relationship. The formal roles and the underlying dimensions (such as the power imbalance, and the expert knowledge of the carer) of those involved exert tremendous influence. They need to be taken into account as the carer–patient relationship develops. How the relationship is set up and framed at the start is a crucial psychological consideration. For example, to what extent do (or will) the parties have shared information, or access to it. Are there dependency considerations to consider? Are all the parties free to exercise their will, and will the decisions of one affect the future standing or state of being of another? These are just a few of the psychological questions that arise in professional caring relationships and which will affect the dynamic processes at work.

We do not know and cannot be fully aware of all these dynamics. The tendency is to rely on what we do know to guide our actions. The result is that we invariably have to function with an *explicit* relationship structure (the roles, the procedures etc.) in the forefront of our thinking and action. But we must also recognize that there will be an *implicit* structure (covering the dynamics, feelings etc.) affecting what goes on between carers and patients, of which we are not totally aware.

Sometimes an attempt is made to make the relationship very explicit through a well formalized framework of relationship expectations such as between a teacher and a pupil. But in many other cases this relationship structure is less explicit and more variable. Ambiguity of such an important matter can be problematic unless boundaries are introduced and maintained in a rigorous, albeit informal way.

What other formalized relationships come into mind apart from those of teacher–pupil and patient–nurse? Make a note on Fig. 7.22; you may also want to look at my list in Fig. 7.33 for comparison.

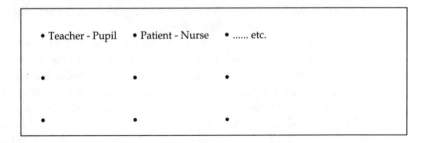

Fig. 7.22   Types of formalized relationships.

I think that attending to the nature and the framing of relationships is very important because this sets out the basis on which:

- subsequent inter-actions occur,
- problems arise,
- expectations are based,
- fantasies are founded,
- trust develops.

What is at the heart of the differences between the types of relationships you have noted in Fig. 7.22? I think a great deal centres around two main dimensions, the first being *expertise* and the second revolving around who *directs the action*. They are both about the exercise of influence and about power. If they are combined we end up with a framework that can be used to contrast the different types of relationship that arise as these two variables change (see Fig. 7.24 for an example). Figure 7.23 indicates what I mean.

Different Combinations	Description	Characteristic
#1 High Expert & High Self Directed	expert, self-directed	autonomy
#2 High Expert & Low Self Directed	expert, passive	unfocused
#3 Low Expert & High Self Directed	active companion	engaged, alert
#4 Low Expert & Low Self Directed	passive passenger	lost, aimless

Fig. 7.23 Two dimensions underpinning relationships.

I do not know how you would characterisze the four different combinations above but I have hazarded a guess. You may wish to select different descriptions for your own use. The main point is to explore the impact which the different combinations of expertise and personal direction have on the type of relationship.

Patients need, and look, for guidance and direction from those who are knowledgeable. These are usually their doctors and nurses, whose directives they are usually prepared to follow as instructed. After a brief period of adjustment and re-orientation however, the patient (depending on their condition) is likely to want to reassert themself in their new surroundings. They want to move from 'low expert and low self-direction' ((4) in Fig. 7.23) type of relationship with others to some other type. While still dependent on others for their expertise and care, the patient may seek to alter the relationship to (3). This allows him to have a say, become more actively involved with care staff and become more involved in his own therapy and treatment.

This model also suggests that the patient is unlikely to be able to move to level (1) or (2), given that they are in need of direct care, however much they may want this. However, allowing the patient, where clinically possible and appropriate, to move from (4) to (3) and for professional staff to move from (2) to (1) is desirable for both patient care and recovery. It also reduces some of the stress and pressure on professional staff caught in the doctor–patient and expert–novice patterns.

In Fig. 7.24 I have used these two dimensions to illustrate some of the variations possible. This offers you another way of thinking about the variable nature of the nurse–patient relationship. Power, influence, dependency, and autonomy are likely to be on the minds of patients and staff. One way of getting to grips with these preoccupations is to think more directly about the impact they can have on behaviour at work and to have a straightforward way of considering what the effect of different balances of *expertness* and *direction* can be.

I have used the dimensions 'expert professional–passive follower' and 'directed by others–self-directed' as a way of discussing the different types of position people can occupy when these two characteristics are put together to different degrees (see Fig. 7.24). The purpose of these ideas is to generate discussion and not to be used as a way of pigeon-holing a person. It is likely that we can occupy positions at either end of the two dimensions I have used, which will depend on what is being done and who else is there at that time.

So with these caveats in mind look at the four different cases below. How would you describe a person with these ways of working? By contrasting these two dimensions you can get a clue as to the likely approach that person is taking at this time. This can help you to understand their position and then to try to work with them more appropriately. This can be done either by encouraging them to become more engaged and active, or by helping them to realize they cannot become the sole directors and experts on the care they need to receive

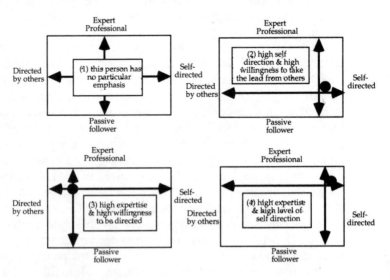

Fig. 7.24 Some ideas about diagnosing relationship styles.

etc. It can give you a quick sense of a person and if there is any benefit in trying to encourage them to relate differently to you.

When you think about your relationship with patients in these terms where do you mainly position yourself along these two dimensions? Do you find that you invariably stick to a constant pattern, or do you find it more productive to change the expert and directed balance? On what criteria do you make such a judgement? Do you show flexibility based on the needs of the patient, or on your own needs at that time? It is worth asking yourself the question since this may help you be clearer about what you do, why and when.

From your experience, and from your readings, what do you consider we need from (or in) our relationships with others? What do we give in return? More clarity here will help you to assess patient needs in this regard and allow you to become clearer about the type of relationships you may prefer.

The following list offers some of my thoughts for you to consider. They illustrate themes I see that underlie people's behaviour and relationships with others. The most common seem to involve the following types of relationships and interactions:

- giving or taking
- selling or buying,
- custodial or protective,
- directing or receiving,
- developmental or remedial,
- collaborative.

In Fig. 7.25 I have shown these in the form of a clockface and would like you to consider what types of interactions seem to underpin your relationships with others. Each diagram has the relationship dimensions I have noted above. On the left diagram mark for each dimension how

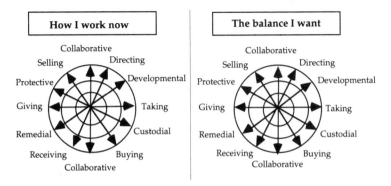

Fig. 7.25 Defining the basis of my relationships with others.

often you notice if you work from that basis in your relations (inner ring = a little; middle ring = often; outer ring = generally the basis from which I work most of the time). With the two 'collaborative' ends I expect them to have the same extension from the centre of the clockface.

What you will now have is a series of marks on each of the 12 points. See what profile has emerged based on your view of the basis on which you work currently. Now think if there are any changes or shifts in emphasis you would like to make. Use the figure on the right to indicate how you would like it to be in the future. The two profiles will now highlight areas of difference. You can think whether or not these changes are appropriate for the work you do; appropriate for the care needed for your patients; and congruent with your own values about what is important to you. I have included a work example of this in Fig. 7.33.

Use these thoughts to note the ways you can start to make any changes you believe to be desirable and beneficial.

You may find that completing Fig. 7.26 will help you to draw into more focus how you prefer to work with others and what you may now need to start doing if you want to work differently in the future. On the other hand, you may have decided that having made them more explicit, you prefer to leave your current ways of working as they are.

The Change I want to make	Why this is important	First steps	What would Help... / Hinder..

Fig. 7.26   Thoughts about changes and how I relate to others.

Special care relationships – living with loss: a challenge and a threat

Every relationship with a client and a patient is important yet it can be easy to forget this or discount the intensity involved for a number of reasons. In part it may be done to protect yourself from the strain of living in such a highly charged setting day after day. It may be because of the growing familiarity, the routinization of care that imposes itself after a time. It may be because of other matters of importance to you that are on your mind. The end result though is the same. There is a possibility that the patient becomes more of an animated object to be cared for and less of an individual to be worked with. This happens.

Yet there remain many conditions where the quality of the nursing care is of continuing, paramount importance. Also where the severity, the prognosis and/or the inequity of the patient's condition impacts on the care providers. This is particularly so with nurses in ways which make the work emotionally exhausting and psychologically demanding. Many cases revolve around living with, and through, loss.

This aspect of a nurse's relationship with patients is particularly difficult because, whilst it originates in the patient, it also touches the nurse in a deeply profound way. It awakens the nurse's own experiences of beginnings, endings, of a hope for continuity, and of mortality. Being able to contend with these issues and stay focused on the caring work in hand, with composure, compassion and care, demands a great deal from the nurse.

From her extensive work with the dying, Kubler-Ross (1970) has identified several stages of adaptation experienced by many patients. She has proposed five stages of adjustment through which the dying patient may pass in their adaptation to their new awareness:

● First stage: denial and isolation
● Second stage: anger
● Third stage: bargaining
● Fourth stage: depression
● Fifth stage: acceptance.

She notes too that throughout this whole process the patient usually maintains a hope for some curative reprieve, not in the sense of a denial but rather the possibility that their recovery may still just occur.

Parkes (1972) from his work with the bereaved has identified five stages often experienced by those suffering from bereavement. He describes them as:

> (1) *Alarm* leading
> to (2) *Searching*
> to (3) *Mitigation*
> to (4) *Anger and guilt*
> towards (5) *Gaining a new identity.*

Parkes notes that apart from grief two other factors always play a part in determining the overall reaction to a bereavement. These are *stigma* and *deprivation*.

> By stigma I mean the change of attitude that takes place in society when a person dies and deprivation implies the absence of a necessary person or thing as opposed to a loss of that person or thing. A bereaved person reacts to both loss and deprivation.

These patterns of personal reaction and change by Kubler-Ross and Parkes offer ways for the nurse to consider more comprehensively the reactions they see from patients who are experiencing a profound psychological sense of loss, perhaps of an earlier sense of certainty in life, and a confusion of where they are now in life. Their work offers insights into the adaptive processes that patients (and nurses too) may pass through in coming to terms with their life following a disruptive or traumatic change.

In Fig. 7.27 I have noted some of the personal losses that give rise to the intense emotional reactions nurses work with and therefore need to be prepared to handle.

LOSS	LOSS	LOSS
• of another	• of independence	• of illusion
• of what could have been	• of self esteem	• of sexuality
• of a job & career	• desired body form	• of health
• of a relationship	• of a partner	• of love
• physical loss	• of reason	• of belief
• of value in the eyes of others	• of meaning and purpose	

Fig. 7.27   Examples of loss.

What other examples of loss would you add to those noted above? The range and variety of stimuli that may induce in us a sense of loss is quite wide and of course this differs for each of us. The whole definition of 'loss' in itself is complex and intensely personal. What I may experience as 'no big deal' could be something of considerable significance for someone else. For example a seemingly uneventful ward event can come to represent major importance. It could be a significant loss to a patient (or a nurse), of which you may be completely unaware at the time only to appreciate later. These types of loss can be carried around internally by patients for some time. They can only be unloaded if you regularly create opportunities for patients to articulate and explore their daily traumas and concerns and thus to begin to discharge them.

In the same way an experience on the ward may profoundly affect you and your work. For colleagues also experiencing that event it may be seen as a matter of little account. They may neither realize how disturbed you were by it or that you may need support and reassurance.

For both the cared-for and the carers there is need for regular opportunities and a collegiate preparedness to review, share and work through such issues and experiences. Being prepared to try to understand each person's perspectives on their concerns as they are being experienced is more constructive and developmental than being told 'it will be all right' or that 'others have felt just as you do now, but they quickly get over it . . .'.

Individual reactions to shock and change

As you will recall from Part Two we are different in how we see things, about what causes us 'angst' and how we respond to the ebbs and flows of life. However, there seem to be common reaction patterns in our personal responses to shock and trauma.

The following are two of these patterns that you can use in your work with patients and for monitoring how you progress. In using these ideas remember that the theory is not that you tell people at what stage they are, but that these are patterns for you to keep in mind. They will help you to support patients and clients appropriately and give you some awareness of the likely next stage of their adaption to their new situation in working through their experiences.

I have found these to be of considerable practical help in reminding me:

- to give others the space and time they need to work things through,
- not to become unduly shocked and dismayed when they turn on me, although it still shakes me to some degree,
- that it is not my job to push them through the cycle,
- I have not failed if they are still having difficulties, so long as I am there to give support, to listen with care and to be there for and with them in their struggle to come to terms with matters.

The time it takes for the sequence to be worked through will vary in each case. For some there may never be a coming to terms with the shock or trauma they have experienced.

The first model in Fig. 7.28, looks at personal adaptation from an organizational perspective. It comes from work with members of organizations going through major changes. From their work Fink *et al.* (1971) (Fig. 7.28) summarized the patterns towards adjustment and personal change into four main reaction stages. They identified some of the related emotions and perspectives which people felt during each stage.

Initially, following trauma, the person is shell-shocked so there is little point in explaining all the details to them. While they may look at you, smile and nod their head they don't know where they are or comprehend all that you are saying. How many times have you explained something to a patient when they are just not ready to comprehend? You may do better to help them through the shock they are experiencing (this could take some time) before you try to do any more.

Reaction Stage	Personal Experience	Orientation to reality	Attitude	Thoughts
1. SHOCK	Threat	Denial	Helplessness Anger	Unwillingness to reason
2. DEFENSIVE RETREAT	Defend	Still too nasty to think about	Cynicism	Planning for subversion
3. ACKNOWL- EDGMENT	Uncomfy & uneasy, but...	Passive adjustment	more open to the possibilities	OK, so tell me what to do...
4. ADAPTATION and CHANGE	Growing sense of security now	Actively engaged	Belief growing again	More positive planning now

Fig. 7.28 Reactions to shock and change.

The table then alerts you to other aspects of their relationship with you during each stage. Of course, there is never any guarantee that they will totally reach a stage of adaptation and acknowledgement of the issues that have impacted upon them. However, you can use this table to guide you as to how they may be feeling and what to watch out for as they comes to terms with everything.

The second approach plots a person's reactions in their level of confidence in themselves and in their ability to see their way through the difficulties, traumas and concerns they experience after a major shock or life event. Following the shock of the event there will often be some denial. This effectively immobilizes the person for a period. They then re-evaluate the situation in terms of some failing on their part. They begin to blame themselves before, however, at the next stage they get angry and focus their anger onto other people and start blaming them.

At this stage their coming to terms has centred primarily around resisting reality. It could be a personal matter for them, the loss of a dear one etc., and this will be a trying period. Now comes the time for trying to come to terms with, and acceptance and acknowledgement of, what has happened. Such a coming to terms with what has transpired offers the possibility of a more productive and problem-solving orientation; a 'good enough' working through of their trauma. Life, or peace of mind, can then be sufficiently re-established to move on from their pre-occupations of the immediate past.

What is never known is how long this will take. Each of us is liable to become stuck at one of these stages or we may find that we oscillate between two of them for a time. Figure 7.29. shows the pattern as a 'big

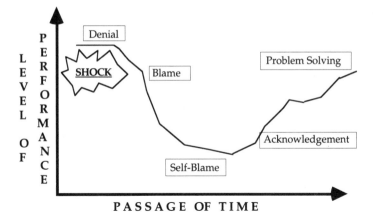

Fig. 7.29 Hopson's response sequence.

dipper' with self-blame as the lowest phase of confidence and effectiveness (Hopson and Hough, 1973). The adaptation and resolution of the trauma then recovers from that low point.

One point to note about both the stages and the sequences outlined above is that once you have gone through some of the stages, it does not mean that you won't necessarily go through them again. Sometimes it only takes a seemingly minor incident to knock you back. You can find yourself worrying about matters you thought you had resolved months, or even years ago. If this happens you must try to help yourself through the process once again. It is the same for your patients. You may see them work through some issue, declare they are all right only to subsequently become preoccupied, perhaps immobilized for a time, with the same issue with which they had previously said they had come to terms. Your psychological care strategy will then be to reinforce their resolve and their intent to work through it once again.

The key message is that each of us is different, not only in how we see things but also in how we respond and react to personal events. You may find it salutary to acknowledge that while you may think that you know what your patients are going through, the best you can do will probably only be a poor approximation. But this means a great deal. When you have been able to appreciate your patient's condition in this way you will have noticed how reassured, touched, grateful – stunned even – your patients have become. That you have got even close to experiencing for yourself their experience is a major accomplishment.

Side effects and surprises

This chapter started by emphasizing the pivotal role occupied by the nurse and how this leads the patient to build up a wide range of expectations of what the nurse can do. When these expectations are not satisfied, or when they are denied by the nurse, these unsatisfied expectations can be converted into negative, possibly abusive, behaviour towards the nurse.

This can mean that one moment the patient is pleasant but then suddenly, almost without notice, they can change to be hostile. This can cause a disarmingly disruptive impact on the carers. Especially during the years of training, this may lead a nurse to wonder if they are competent, capable or careful enough. They may wonder if this really is a profession they are suited to enter and be a part of.

One of the ways we protect ourselves when we experience threat or anxiety is to look at such situations, people and things as being either *good* or *bad*. We then attach good or bad labels to those objects or people depending how we experience them. When we are pleased or disappointed we attribute and attach some of our intense emotional feelings onto other people and onto objects. We give them varying degrees of 'goodness' and/or 'badness' depending whether or not our needs have been satisfied or frustrated.

This is what can happen when a patient's expectations, realistic or not, are met, denied or somehow thwarted. The person they deem responsible for this can then become the focus for their response. This can carry with it an emotional force which can be either positive or negative and out of all proportion to the situation itself.

The nurse can then be considered by the patient as either a 'good' nurse or a 'bad' one. Incidentally, that very same nurse is also likely to be seen by that same patient as both 'good' and 'bad' depending on whether the patient is getting what it wants from them.

What I am referring to is how a patient can generate and then project onto the nurse intense emotional feelings that have come from some deep need which has been met or denied. The emotional impact of these processes on the nurse can be very traumatic. This is even more so if these matters are not recognized or discussed as a difficult and very potent aspect of ward life.

The point is that patients (and others, including ourselves) have a tendency to invest strong emotional feelings onto people and objects. This can have an intensity out of proportion to the matters being handled. When this does happen it does not mean that the nurse is 'good' or 'bad' per se but in order to continue functioning the patient has utilized (unconsciously) these good–bad defences.

This 'splitting' of one's view of a person or of an object into 'good' or 'bad' is an attempt to cope with intense anxieties they are experiencing. In this case they do it through projecting these feelings externally.

Stress awakened – what does it mean for you?

The considerations outlined in this chapter suggest that to remain effective both as a professional carer, and as a person, each nurse needs to handle intense interpersonal dynamics and tensions effectively and efficiently. These are likely to create levels of stress, physical tension and tiredness. Unless acknowledged and worked through, these could lead to a deterioration of the professional quality of the service provided along with emotional and physical dehabilitation of the nurse. This could show itself in different ways including absenteeism, high sickness rates, a lowering of morale and cohesion, organizational tensions and disagreements etc.

Figure 7.30 shows some of the causes and triggers of stress for nurses. What others would you add in and which ones affect you?

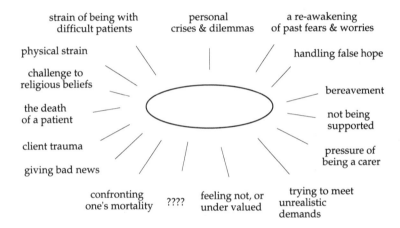

strain of being with difficult patients

personal crises & dilemmas

a re-awakening of past fears & worries

physical strain

handling false hope

challenge to religious beliefs

bereavement

the death of a patient

not being supported

client trauma

pressure of being a carer

giving bad news

confronting one's mortality

????

feeling not, or under valued

trying to meet unrealistic demands

Fig. 7.30 Sources of stress for nurses.

My emphasis in Fig. 7.30 has been on identifying some of the stresses and strains that arise from being a professional carer but there are also those that come from your place in the organization itself. Whether you feel you are in the 'right' job or not (in terms of role, department, speciality, firm, etc.) exert a tremendous influence on your well-being and sense of worth. Generally people try to move into roles in which they feel comfortable and secure. Difficulties arise when there is too big a gap between the role they want to occupy and where they are now, and from situations where they are unable to operate in their role in ways they believe to be professionally appropriate. Tensions and stresses are generated if there is an incongruence between what I want to do, and how I wish to fulfil that role.

Distress is also caused where you are either unable, or not allowed to be, yourself. What does this mean? Can you recall situations (from school, college, home, etc.) when you were told to be like someone else, or where unless you did it like *X* did, what you were doing was not acceptable? How did you feel about that? If you were able to emulate the performance/behaviour of *X* and if you valued them as well, perhaps you didn't mind too much.

If though you were unable to do it the way *X* did, or if *X* was a person you held in particularly low regard, then you may have experienced considerable anxiety and discomfort.

What personal examples of this type of situation can you now recall, from any part of the past? These are recollections of situations where you wanted to respond in a professional manner but you were directed to respond in a manner or a style that was in conflict with your own personal or professional style. It is possible that the guidance you were given was

	Description of the situation	How I wanted to be myself	What I was told to be like	Consequences for me and others
Example 1:				
Example 2:				
Example 3:				

Fig. 7.31   The 'Me'/not 'Me' dilemma.

reasonable and appropriate, but it is also possible that it felt that you were being forced to compromise your own sense of yourself. You were being told to work, act, feel or be different to how you were, irrespective of your professional competence and experience to do the task required.

Such instances can leave you with a feeling of being violated, of not being acceptable as you are. You may have had the feeling of being almost victimized by the other person(s) who may seem to have been trying to get you to be someone you are not. This is stressful and can make you uneasy and perhaps a little confused about your value and worth. It can generate self-doubt and cripple otherwise able people. You will recall from the 'internal conversations' section in Part Two, we each seem to have a tendency to engage in self-doubt.

Stressful and worrying though these instances are it is not always acceptable to show your feelings. Thus they cannot be discussed and worked through with colleagues, and consequently they are often left unattended to. It may be that there is no recognition by anyone else that anything at all was amiss. You may have been told that you had no cause for complaint (or stress) and, therefore, there are no issues to be worked through. This can make your experience even more trying because it has not been validated by others.

Two scenarios come to mind. When this happens you may start to feel a bit low. You may feel more easily tired than before, and you may be surprised to find yourself wondering if nursing really is for you (scenario one). An alternative scenario (scenario two) is that you *are* very aware when you are not allowed to be yourself in undertaking your responsibilities even though you perform them ethically and in a professional manner. In fact you get incensed that someone else should have the gall to tell you what is and what is not acceptable about yourself and you are unwilling to copy someone else.

If it is not possible, or acceptable, to vent and discuss your feelings – so that the matters can be worked through – they will stay with you. If these feelings are not expressed they will fester inside you. In this scenario you are angry, whereas in the first you are more passive and accepting.

In both of these scenarios there is a violation of an acceptance of who you are by others as well as a block to a discussion of how you feel about this. In both cases this is likely to lead to a depowering of your view of yourself and will generate unhelpful levels of stress. Added to this psychological injury you may be in a setting where you are expected not only to 'put a brave face on it' but to 'look happy' and this will add to the strain and sense of neglect you may be feeling. Sometimes you may not be fully aware of such pressures. You just conform, but do so uneasily and with a sense of something not being right or as it should be.

Did you remember learning about magnets at school? You may recall that they have magnetic fields·. Although you cannot actually see them just by looking, when you put a magnet near some iron filings you then see, through the behaviour of the filings within the range of the magnet, the unseen force of the magnet influences the subsequent behaviour of the iron filings. This can be applied to you at work. There are several fields of unseen, emotional influence which nevertheless exercise an influence on your behaviour and your thoughts.

These emotional 'fields' need to be accommodated, adapted to and worked with. They are an integral part of your place of work. Mostly we are unaware of these processes occurring but sometimes we will experience the adaptation we are being asked to make to our behaviour so starkly, that it forces us to notice these pressures. This could happen in a situation where a core value of yours comes under threat, perhaps where you see an injustice occurring and want to do something about it. Another example is where you are reminded of a painful personal experience and you wish, with hindsight, you could have responded differently.

There will be instances where you are aware of the emotional significance of some events or interactions in the present, yet you are blocked institutionally from responding as you would wish. This could be because you have been instructed not to do so, or because of a threat of retribution. As you are grappling with this you may also be required to present a positive face to those around you. If you want to remain in a positive light this will require a denial and suppression of your feelings and emotions.

This is not about emotional outbursts. My focus is on what it feels like when you consider you are being pushed to work in ways that are not in tune with your view of yourself, where you can find yourself caught between being true to yourself or complying with an organizational requirement. It may be ethical and appropriate, but it is not your way.

Hochschild (1983) talks about these pressures and differentiates between what he calls *emotional work* and *emotional labour*. Emotional work is the effort we put into ensuring that our private feelings are suppressed or represented to be in tune with socially accepted norms. Emotional labour is the commercial exploitation of this principle, for example when an employee is 'paid' to smile, laugh, be polite, or 'be caring' but which rests uneasily with a person's underlying forces and tensions which will be seeking unrestricted expression. This can result in increasing internal tension and frustration.

Concluding comments

If you decide that you want your situation to change, then you must decide what you are after and marshal your resources to bring about that change. You will need to let it be known to others what you want, when and how. This is easier said than done. It can be difficult to get the balance right between being assertive about what you want and being considered aggressive. This is especially so if your wants challenge or contest the *status quo*. The next few chapters discuss this and show how for many of us this requires practice, judgement and perseverance.

One consequence of the material covered in this chapter is that while you will not always feel good about things, you will be better equipped to identify why this might be. You will then be able to plan appropriate and sensitive action. Situations on and off the ward may not be as you like all the time, neither are they 'hell on earth' even though they are difficult at times. It is within these limits that we go about our business and work as best we can.

Given the inherent personal challenges of being a nurse it is important to understand the array of pressures and stresses that impinge on you as a carer. To discharge your professional responsibilities with competence and compassion demands that you care sufficiently for yourself. The challenge is being able to keep these two requirements in balance and in mind.

Appendix A: Worked examples

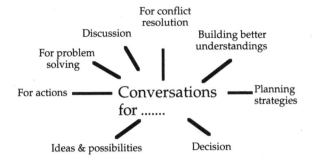

Fig. 7.32 A worked example for Fig. 7.3.

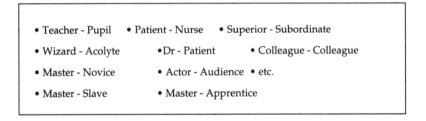

Fig. 7.33 A worked example for Fig. 7.22.

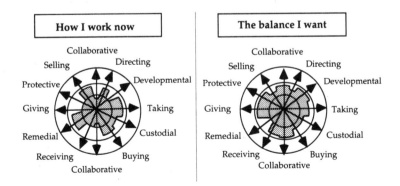

Fig. 7.34 A worked example for Fig. 7.25.

References

Argyle, M. (1967) *The Psychology of Interpersonal Behaviour*, Penguin, Harmondsworth.

Fink, S. *et al.* (1971) Organizational crisis and change *The Journal of Applied Behavioural Science* **7.1**.

Hochschild, A. (1983) *The Managed Heart*, University of California Press, Berkeley, USA.

Hopson, B. and Hough, P. (1973) *Exercises in Personal and Career Development*, Careers Research, Cambridge.

Kubler-Ross, E. (1970) *On Death and Dying*, Tavistock Publications, London.

Menzies, I. (1970) *The Functioning of Social Systems as a Defence Against Anxiety*. Tavistock Institute of Human Relations, London.

Parkes, C. (1972) *Bereavement: Studies of Grief in Adult Life*, Tavistock Publications, London.

Further reading

Charles-Edwards, D. (1992) *Counselling Issues of Managers No 1: Death Bereavement and Work*, CEPEC, London.

Fineman, S. (1993) *Emotion in Organizations*, Sage Publications, London.

Madders, J. (1988) *Stress and Relaxation*, Macdonald Optima, London.

Owens, R. and Naylor, F. (1989) *Living while Dying*, Thorsons, Wellingborough.

Parkinson, F. (1993) *Post-Trauma Stress*, Sheldon Press, London.

Shepherd, E. (1994) *Becoming Skilled*, The Law Society, London.

Chapter 8
Working with Others

What is involved and why it is difficult to achieve

The purpose of this chapter is to cover some methods you can use to get a better grip on influencing others. Also how to stand up for yourself, enhance the quality of communication with others and how to handle conflict at work. Some of the material overlaps with material elsewhere in the book and you may want to draw on that additional material from time to time.

I have gone for straightforward ideas about these topics so that you will be able to keep them in mind and use them where appropriate. I believe that if you can make more sense of what is going on then you will have a better opportunity of remaining effective in situations that otherwise could swamp you. You don't want to get swamped too often. It doesn't do you much good, and you cannot care for others very effectively either.

We all need to work with others, yet at the same time it is very difficult to do so. We have our own wants and priorities and these can be very different from those around us. We want to collaborate and be friendly, yet we have a need to keep our own counsel and be independent. If you sometimes wonder why you have problems in getting on with others it may not necessarily be your fault. It could be the difficulty that most of us have, wanting to be part of, yet at the same time different from others.

Keep in mind the work you completed in Part Two. Being sensitive to your needs and goals is essential in becoming more effective in your work with others. It also helps you to realize why some of the differences may be arising. If you have a low opinion of your capabilities and are unaware of your potential then you will find it very difficult to influence others around you. They may like you a lot but they may not take you seriously. You will not come over in a focused way as a person who believes in themself, has ideas about their future intentions and who can be respected.

Taking yourself seriously is one point but you also need to take seriously your working relationships with others. You can do this by drawing on some more ideas and frameworks about interpersonal relations.

135

What I need to take into account when working with others

Setting aside individual differences for the moment. Fig. 8.1 sets out a number of additional features that are present in any interaction and which influence the course, nature and results from that interaction. These are:

(1) the issues explicitly presented for consideration,
(2) where the meeting takes place,
(3) the background and history surrounding the meeting/interaction itself,
(4) the unexpected issues and concerns that are also in the meeting of both those which are known – but which nobody is talking about – as well as unconscious ones.

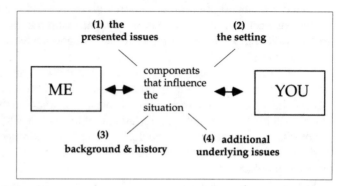

Fig. 8.1   Key features in an interaction.

(1) The presented issues

The common ground between all present is the formally declared purpose for the meeting. For example, to agree the new shift pattern, or to agree on the care strategy for a patient, or perhaps to write the proposal for a change in bed use. However the formal agenda does not include all the relevant material. Sometimes people will withhold or misrepresent relevant material. Sometimes critical issues are unable to be worked on because no-one is able to express them well enough.

The presented issues are the formally presented care and business matters that require attention. These include the items on the agenda, those we know we are there to work on and on which we are expected to have views, data and opinions.

(2) The setting

Where and how we meet significantly influences the tone and style of the interactions and can influence what will be achievable. Choosing the setting is a strategic decision. It should not be left to chance if there are a range of options from which to select. It can make all the difference for example, if the meeting is on neutral ground or in the boss's office, if it is in the district general hospital or in the school, etc. The time of day is another important factor. You are likely to get better quality interactions and decisions if you hold your meeting at a mutually convenient time, and have set aside the time you need.

(3) The background and history to your contact

Each person present brings with them their own personal history. This includes their wider aspirations, their strengths and their areas of weakness, all of which they will utilize in one way or another in their interactions with you. Each person also brings with them a history of earlier dealings with you or your department, expectations based on their assessment of the past and what they think will now transpire.

Taking account of the historical perspective is often neglected yet this can give clues about what is likely to happen in the current meeting. We build up a track history of each other through working directly with each other. Through our network of contacts we build up an idea of what people we have yet to work with are like. In such ways we put history and our imagination to work. We are unlikely to meet new colleagues 'cold' because, if we can, we collect views about them from others beforehand, we see what the track record suggests and then plan accordingly.

Much of this is about trust and regard, and we look to the past to see what we can predict for the future.

(4) Additional underlying issues and considerations

These are the additional agenda issues which are there in the interactions but not formally acknowledged; often called the hidden agenda. There are also the underlying dynamics and tensions that will be generated during the interactions. Much of this is likely to be stimulated by unconscious communications.

All of these dimensions come together and exert influence on what takes place. Because of the unknown composition of the mix of influences created, this makes the detailed course of many meetings and interactions unpredictable.

You can apply these ideas to what happens when you and your colleagues work together, to you working with your patients, and to settings outside work. You can start by thinking of an interaction that is likely to take place shortly. Use Fig. 8.1 to speculate – for each person expected to be there – on the views they might hold about the issues to be considered. What are the underlying issues (irrespective of the formal purpose set for the meeting)? What is the effect of the proposed setting for the meeting, and what has happened when you have met previously?

What history and background of hospitals, clinics, home visits etc., might your patients bring with them that will affect and influence their behaviour with you and your colleagues. Do they hold the view that you only go to hospital as a last resort? Do they have a view that they will not be told anything, or that they will be bullied and be made to do unpleasant things? What stories have they been told – good as well as bad – about your hospital? These will condition how they interact with you.

If you think about *settings* patients will have different reactions depending where they are located. Being located in a small four bedded room rather than a large 20 bedded open ward for example, will give quite different care experiences, irrespective of the actual clinical care delivered. The state of the decor will affect things too. It could both reassure and frighten them if the decor is too clinical. Some facilities may be unfamiliar to them and cause them confusion and distress. Some features – like a day room – may cause great pleasure. Perhaps for the first time for many years they have been part of a 'family' sitting around watching the television, whereas for others it may be something to be avoided at all costs because of past memories.

There is a view that behind every question there is a statement being made. When a patients asks you something (*the presented issue*) is there another unstated question or a statement that they are making to you (*the underlying issue*) that needs teasing out and addressing? To tease these out takes effort, attention and an awareness of your own, and of the other person's needs. If you are to build and sustain friendships and collaborative working relationships you will need to be aware of this. This is not easy to achieve. Each time you meet, intervening experiences may have caused both of you to see certain things differently to before. This could lead you to view that particular relationship rather differently as well.

Since we are sensitive to human experiences you could, as part of your clinical approach, remain alert for signals in yourself and from others that something has altered or is in the process of changing between you. It is probably not surprising that some of the most commonly used greetings between people are along the lines of 'How are you doing . . . ?' or 'So what's new . . . ?' or 'Everything OK . . . ?' These are our ritualized ways of checking the state of each other. The sad news is that these greetings of enquiry so often become rhetorical questions, where the expected and desired response is 'Fine thank you' rather than a genuine invitation to engage. It can be like a pointless ritual where you both make a noise to each other before getting on with your work, uninterested and unaffected by whatever reply was given.

This is why some people get very anxious and uncomfortable when, in response to the ritual question, you do actually tell them how you are and about some of your current difficulties etc. Perhaps there should be a rule that says 'Don't ask the question unless you really want to know – because if you ask me I may decide to tell you!' See what happens when you respond fully next time to the neighbour who says 'Hello, all right then?'

In your work with patients and colleagues you could use the format of Fig. 8.2 to remind yourself to take into account the shared background of experiences as a backdrop to current priorities and also to consider the desired future you are working towards.

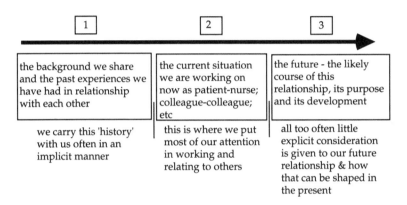

Fig. 8.2 Working from the past to look into the future.

Changing relationships

In the main we don't give adequate attention to the regular, repetitive interactions we have with those we know. We proceed on the basis of 'it will be the same as last time'. At times it clearly is not the same and that is when we are most likely to over-react, misread or are shocked by what happens. We can be defensive, possibly aggressive, as a reaction to the unexpected difficulty we experience with someone we thought we knew, and someone who was 'safe' for us.

You may recall cases where what began as just another regular ward handover meeting, or evening drugs round, or a comment to the team member suddenly became something else that you were not prepared for and just as suddenly became far reaching in its consequences.

A good point to remember is that however it may appear, the relationship with someone else is rarely fixed for ever. It will continue to move and develop all the time. While certain patterns and interactional sequences become formalized between people and come to occupy an important part of any relationship there will always remain the possibility of a major change that could fundamentally alter the *status quo* you have come to expect, and even depend upon.

The following dimensions in Fig. 8.3 need to be considered in building and maintaining relationships. You will have a lot of information about some of these but will only be able to speculate about others such as unexpressed needs from the relationships. But doing this type of review will help you to remain sensitive to changes in your working relationships.

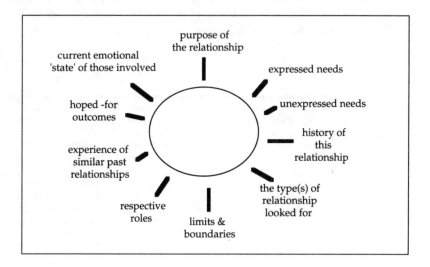

Fig. 8.3 Remaining sensitive to changes in my relationships with others.

How do I come across?

Before I introduce any more material can you first complete this next exercise in Fig. 8.4. I want you to make a quick summary of how you see yourself and how you are viewed by others. If you wish you can use some of the notes from Part Two. On the other hand you can jot down a few key thoughts about yourself now without trying to cover all the work you did earlier. Please integrate that material later.

Prompted by your notes and using Fig. 8.5, what would you identify as the strong and the weaker points that come out about you? With your notes in mind use the following framework in Fig. 8.6 to extend your notes and to identify a little more fully how your view of yourself might be similar and/or different to a colleague's view of you. This works best if you have a particular person in mind and if you work quite quickly in building up their possible view of you. You may like to do the same with a couple of other people so you end up with a range of three or four views. Concentrate on the 'Others' view of me' column first, then after

---

(a) How I see myself

-
-
-

Now please do the same but working from what others tend to say about you.

(b) How others see me

-
-
-

Fig. 8.4 How I come across to others.

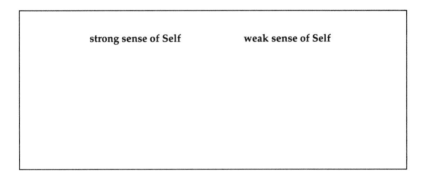

Fig. 8.5 My stronger and weaker points.

you have done this with a few colleagues put in the notes you did about yourself.

You can use this exercise on its own or you might want to use material from Chapter 4, which concentrated on thinking about yourself, and see what new insights emerge. It is very difficult to ascertain how others see you. While it is possible to speculate on their views, you may be quite inaccurate in impressions you recorded above. One possibility is to ask some of your colleagues if they would be prepared to give you some of their views about you. If you do this you may like to give them some headings as a guide, or a copy of one of the diagrams from the book around which to structure their thoughts.

Now compare the messages you are picking up. Firstly, what are

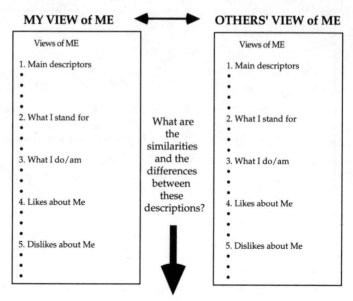

PULLING THESE DIFFERENT PERSPECTIVES TOGETHER

Surprises; Confirmations, Differences, Challenges, Confusions etc etc

Fig. 8.6   Comparing perspectives about myself.

the similarities and differences between your view of you and the views your colleagues have? You can either ask them as suggested above and/or speculate what you anticipate their views to be. How different – and in what ways – are the views expressed? If you did ask colleagues to fill in comments about you how consistent are the responses from them? Do they each see you differently? If they differ a lot, why is that? These are the types of question to use to get the most from the work. The whole idea is that you can become as clear as possible about how you come across to others and the type of impact you have on them.

If colleagues gave you their feedback you can also assess how accurate you were in their views of you. This will give you more food for thought. You can get an idea about how realistic, or perhaps idealistic you are about yourself.

It is worth exploring further:

- where you and others agree about you,
- where there is a difference in perceptions,
- why that may be,
- what attributes are noted,
- what attributes are not noted at all,

- what overall messages come to you,
- if they are the messages you want,
- if they are messages you do not want.

You can summarize the results under the four areas of Fig. 8.7.

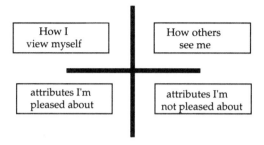

Fig. 8.7 Four important areas to attend to.

There can be a huge difference between what you expect to hear and what is actually said about you. I still get a shock when I find out that there is a discrepancy between how I thought I presented myself and received feedback to the contrary. It blows apart my false perceptions and gives me messages and surprises I had not expected! At least, when I have pondered on it for a while, I have the opportunity to review what I do and reassess my behaviour to make any changes that I feel are needed. If I don't keep myself open to such feedback and retain my ability to reflect on myself, then there is a risk I will become out of touch over time with myself and others as well.

The Johari window

The ability to build effective working relationships and mutual understandings was seen from studies in the late 1960s, to centre around providing *feedback* to others and being prepared to *review and disclose* more information about oneself. The two main sources of information that emerged as important were:

(1) *what I know about myself:* this covers the data about me that is there in the public domain *and* what I know about me that I choose to keep to myself,
(2) *what others know about me:* that I don't!

These ideas were put together by two social psychologists, Joe Ingram and Harry Luft, into a compact framework they called the Johari window as illustrated in Fig. 8.8. Combining the two dimensions creates four different interpersonal scenarios:

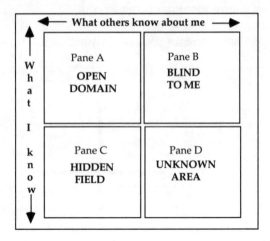

Fig. 8.8 The Johari window.

(1) *Pane A: The open domain:* that contains information about me of which I am very much aware. This would cover things like age band, education, role, interests stated, accent, physical features, musical tastes, expressed views on things, etc. Material, for example, that you and I could easily put down together on paper about me.

(2) *Pane B: Blind area:* in addition to the shared material, other people will see, and grasp things about me that I do not know about. It could be relevant and important for me to know, but it can only come from other people if they choose to tell me.

(3) *Pane C: The hidden field:* in this area could be all sorts of things ranging from my deepest views on matters of great importance to me, which I want to keep to myself, to thoughts about the job and my future career, etc. This is material that I know and could share if I choose to.

Finally, there is a part of me that is available to neither me nor anyone else – the unknown:

(4) *Pane D: The unknown area:* in which there are additional facets of me of which I am not aware, even though they exert an influence on my behaviour and well-being.

Working well with others rests a great deal on the quality of the communications between people and on the quality of the mutual understandings that have been established. One way of doing this is to broaden and deepen the area of common ground between colleagues. This is likely to lead to greater mutual understanding and, possibly, collaboration.

The Johari window suggests two ways in which to achieve this greater mutual understanding. To begin with you need to release more information about yourself that is relevant to the situations you are working in with others. Here you can make a choice to expand the area of Pane A through disclosing material from Pane C.

This may trigger the second way towards more mutual understanding. This is when colleagues feel able to give you constructive feedback: that is data about you that they know but which you are unaware of (from Pane B). Through the processes of *disclosure* and *feedback* you can significantly enlarge the area of the common ground – Pane A – and establish a more open basis on which to work and relate to others.

The way the approach can be used with another person is shown in Fig. 8.9. What you try to achieve is a larger area of shared knowledge between you and the other person. This comes initially from you disclosing something from your hidden area (Pane C) and by showing a willingness to receive some feedback from the other person. By doing this you reduce the size of your blind area – Pane B. You offer a willingness to provide feedback to the other person too and hope that in turn they will also tell you a little more about themselves from their hidden area (Pane C).

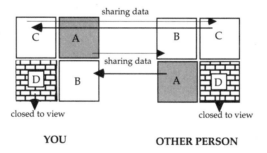

Fig. 8.9   Using the Johari window to build more interpersonal communication and understandings.

Through these two complementary processes of disclosure and receiving feedback, a more robust and soundly based working relationship can, over time, be established. It creates a wider area of shared understanding and trust between the parties involved.

You can now use the information you have elicited from those around you, together with your reflections on yourself to see what messages come out when you put it all together. You may like to consider using the format in Fig. 8.10 to do this and see what comes.

	What evidence do I have for this?	What 'sense' do I make of this
1. What seems to make me tick?		
2. What do I appear to avoid?		
3. What worries, disturbs me?		
4. What to change & what to reinforce?		

Fig. 8.10   Building another view of myself.

Make a note somewhere private and safe of the principal outcomes and messages about yourself that have emerged from this. What implications do you see them having:

- for you as a person,
- for you as a nurse,
- for those you care for,
- for other people more generally?

It may be that little has emerged yet, so do not worry. More will come later.

Unhelpful relationships

The emphasis so far has been on enhancing positive beneficial communications with others, especially patients. This is not the complete story. The potential always exists for the negative and exploitative aspects of human nature to exert their influence, particularly in settings where there are dependent relationships, such as in health care.

Acknowledging that there are influences, motives and intentions that are not always motivated by good is one way of countering their power and influence. It is better than pretending that they don't exist or that you have never had negative thoughts, etc. The potential for misdoing goes hand in hand with our potential for good works and there is always work to be done to keep these two conflicting pulls in balance.

The purpose of this short section is to draw attention to these considerations. Also to highlight some of the ways in which you may develop inappropriate and unhelpful patient/colleague relationships and to show how easy it is for these changes to happen in all of us. Over time exploitative relationships can occur and lead to a situation where what was previously unacceptable behaviour becomes the norm. Examples of this would include:

- being physically and mentally abusive to patients,
- withholding patient benefits,
- exploiting patient dependency for sexual, monetary or informational advantage,
- misuse or misapplication of medication or clinical procedures,
- neglect,
- the exploitative use of the privileged nursing role.

While the exploitation of patients was the main concern, some of the above abuses can be directed onto colleagues and others. To do this requires several features to be in place, such as:

- some type of dominant:less-dominant relationship (see earlier material on models of relationships and expectations),
- the opportunity to exercise authority,
- an intended exploitative reward that will accrue to the dominant person,
- some degree of privacy or protection from public view of what is going on (this can be through a cover-up).

This is by no means an exhaustive list but exploitative relationships rarely happen 'just like that'. There have to be features that support the continuation of abuse in some way. Some institutionalized protection of the abuser is an example, and denial or diminution of the abused person's ability to draw attention to their plight.

Breaking cycles of misconduct and patient abuse is very difficult to achieve. This is partly due to the guilt which the perpetrators will generally experience. They will take self-protective measures and fear the outrage that would follow the knowledge of their activities. Increasingly, however, the subject of the misuse of carer privilege is receiving more coverage in the press. These previously taboo areas are now receiving more widespread attention. The ethical behaviour of the nurse, and the doctor, has always been a topic for debate but the extent to which abuse occurs has been documented rather less.

The dynamics of work groups, notions of group cohesion and of peer group bonding, while positive in many respects, can also make it very difficult for a person to speak out about any worries, doubts or suspicions they may have about patient, or carer, abuse.

Figure 8.11 contrasts positive, developmental and ethical practice on the left-hand side with some of the ways in which the trust gained with a patient can become either dysfunctional or misused by the carer (right-hand side). It may not even be the carer's intention to foster an unethical relationship but over time a dysfunctional one can develop. One way of reducing this possibility is to acknowledge the potential for misuse of trust and to put in place a monitoring system to guard against this.

Responsive Listening	Taking over the patient
An ear to listen with respect and consideration	Rescuing the patient
	Over identification
Creating a climate care & trust	Losing the 'neutral' external perspective
	Misusing the trust given
Enabling options to be raised & considered by the patient	Fuelling fantasy
	Giving the definitive advice

Fig. 8.11   From trusting to exploitive relationships.

The underlying dynamics seem to be:

- growing emotional dependency by the patient on the carer,
- an increasing sense of power by the carer over the patient,
- professional security of the carer in contrast to the relative frailty and weak power base of the patient,
- reducing belief in patient protests when contrasted with the expressed, or taken for granted, professional integrity of the carer.

Differences, disagreements and assertion

One of the most consuming of life's challenges is our ability to get on with other people. While we cannot get on without other human beings, we cannot get on very well with them either. Yet a priority for each of us is to establish effective cooperation. It is one of our major tasks.

Working with others always carries with it concerns about:

- rivalry,
- competition,
- collaboration,
- hope,

- anxiety,
- envy,
- jealousy,
- fantasy,
- seduction,
- validation,
- greed,
- pleasure,
- rage,
- fury
- ecstasy,
- love,
- hate,
- fear.

The list may look a bit fierce, but it covers the raw human emotions which we bring with us into our work with others. Some of these are rarely seen, but they are part of our make-up and they can be triggered from time to time at work. We can find ourselves nudged into competitive win–lose situations which mainly we would prefer not to lose. Some of the intense emotions noted above will be triggered by our feelings of competition or from a sense of frustration that our wants are being thwarted. In such situations it is so easy to become fixated on the need not to lose that we can find ourselves going for a win. By disregarding the consequences we forget that there are other resolution options available, where each of the parties involved can achieve a positive, or 'good enough', outcome.

What can help is to consider what other options are possible but first of all, why do such difficulties occur when we try to work with others? What are differences and disagreements about? Why do you think difficulties occur when people work together? What is it that seems to get in the way? Can you think about some of your recent examples and jot down why you think difficulties arose (see Fig. 8.12)?

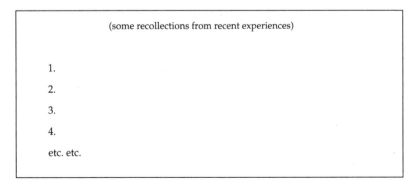

Fig. 8.12 Things that get in the way of working effectively with others.

Now see if there are any common themes or patterns that underlie your examples. Problems may have arisen because of some rivalry that you noticed which got in the way, but what was that rivalry about? It could have been about power, about your personal standing in the eyes of others, or for some other reason. Alternatively the difficulties could have been triggered by professional competition, perhaps because of a lack of trust, or due to differences about the philosophy of care to be followed. See what could underpin and explain the notes you have made above.

Some of the reasons why I believe we experience difficulties in relating to each other are shown in Fig. 8.13. The list is not exhaustive, so you will probably want to add more items that occur to you.

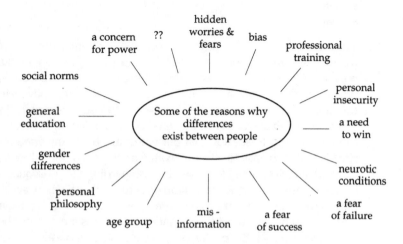

Fig. 8.13 Some reasons why differences exist . . .

Sometimes the problems come from simple misunderstandings. This can be compounded by an organizational belief that its not alright to ask a question or to challenge, even in a constructive way, a decision that most see as inappropriate but against which no one is prepared to take a stand. Sometimes the problems are caused by talking at cross purposes without realizing it. On other occasions the difficulties are rooted in neurotic conditions found in one of the people involved.

Talking at cross purposes

Sometimes difficulties arise because we are not talking on the same wavelength to each other. This can happen when we are not listening carefully enough to the other person. We interpret their lack of agreement as a disagreement, whereas they may only be trying to understand what we are talking about. One way out of this unhelpful cross-purpose communication is to ask the other person to clarify what they are saying. For example, are they talking about *how* we should do it or *when*? Are they emphasizing the *strategy* we should follow or the *sequence* of detailed steps needed? Simple confusions, but hard to detect when each party is concentrating on getting their point across. They are looking for agreement with their point of view, not further clarification or explanation!

It may be that what appear at first sight to be conflicting positions are only different shades of opinion. For example, it is very likely that we will start to disagree with each other if you want to explore the overall strategy and I want to talk about the detailed steps we need to take! We need to realize that we are talking about different aspects of the issue, both of which need attention.

If you can clarify that this is what is taking place then the remedy is to define the various aspects which need to be discussed and then plan to cover all the facets. I have been in top management teams where tensions have risen to a very high degree because of vehement disagreements. They then realize, with some embarrassment, that they were actually agreeing on what should be done, yet talking at cross purposes. They were talking about different aspects of the same thing! When they stopped trying to get their own way they realized there was no substantive disagreement between them at all.

As an example, Fig. 8.14 sets out six different dimensions, each of which is important and needs attention in the explanation and discussion of a proposed action or proposal. Unless each of these different

What **I** am talking about!		What **you** are talking about!
•	(1) the **PHILOSOPHY** of it all	•
•	(2) the **STRATEGY** we should follow	•
•	(3) the **TACTICS** to adopt	•
•	(4) the **RESOURCES** we need	•
•	(5) the **TIMING** to go for	•
•	(6) what **SEQUENCE** to follow	•

Fig. 8.14 Levels of discussion and planning.

considerations are explored, it is likely that any decisions made will not be as soundly based as they should be. Consequently problems may arise in the future through not attending to one or more of these levels. You do not though, in every meeting, need to look at each level – so long as they are covered at some stage.

I have shown them in a hierarchy for two reasons. The first is to indicate that you need to be clear about the philosophy of what you are doing. Then you can decide on other areas like strategy and the timing of actions. At the top of my hierarchy is the underlying philosophy and the rest follows in the sequence shown. The second reason is to show that if you can identify what people are talking about, you can then use this diagram to illustrate how you are focusing on different considerations and what considerations have been missed.

In the figure I have illustrated how you can determine where you and a colleague may be focusing attention in the discussion of a piece of work.

Can you think back to a recent situation where there were difficulties in reaching some agreements or shared understandings? Could you have used this framework to identify at what level those involved were concentrating on exploring the issues under consideration? Did any of the problems or tensions you experienced, or observed, arise because there were these types of 'crossed wires'? Were people talking very earnestly, but at different levels of this hierarchy and just 'missing' each other's contributions? If so you now have a way of reducing the likelihood of this happening in the future.

Conflicts at work

Sometimes no matter how you might seek to avoid it you find yourself in a situation of conflict. The choices open to you then are *how* to respond. Perhaps the most basic response you may consider is whether to fight and get involved or to do the opposite and flee from it (the fight–flight response). Sometimes you may have no option but to take one of these. Sometimes the most prudent and constructive approach is to move away from the situation if you assess that there is little to be gained by staying involved and fighting it out. There are though other options available to you that are not so black and white and which are not so risky for the people involved.

The first step is to try to identify what is causing the conflict in the first place. If you can select three recent examples, can you make a note of what you consider was at the heart of those difficulties? Make a note of these in Fig. 8.15. What were the conflicts about?

Here are some thoughts from my experience of reasons for conflicts at work:

- competing bids for power and influence
- strong win–lose culture

Recent examples of conflict situations	What was causing the difficulties?
•	•
•	•
•	•

Fig. 8.15 Clarifying the cause of recent conflicts.

- personality clashes
- clash of values
- lack of a shared view of the problem to be tackled
- professional politics
- professional rivalry
- maintaining 'face' and credibility
- disagreements about what to do
- no shared goals
- do not have the same information
- mistrust
- self-protection and covering up.

These are just a few and no doubt you have others to add to this list. Try to look beneath the conflict to see why it is happening and what it is all about. If you can do this there may be ways to either move things onto a more constructive footing or, at least, to look for ways of reducing some of the animosity that may be present.

There are two prime considerations to take account of when working with conflict. The first is to reach a position where you satisfy your objectives. The second is to avoid destroying the relationships with those with whom you have the conflict. While this will not always be possible to achieve, common sense dictates that it is of little value for you to win the battle only to jeopardize your future working relationships with key colleagues.

Thomas (1976) identified five major styles of conflict management which he developed into a very useful model. Figures 8.16 and 8.17 are based on his work. Thomas suggests five main styles that can be used to resolve conflicts and to negotiate outcomes, each of which have their advantages and their limitations. Each style represents a different balance between being assertive and being cooperative.

It may be that each of these styles has a different appeal to you. You

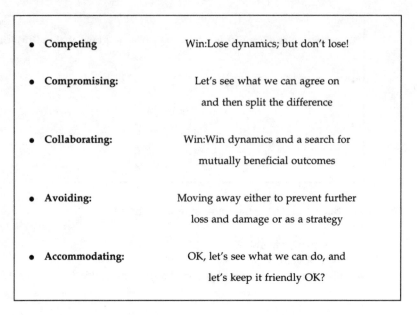

- **Competing**   Win:Lose dynamics; but don't lose!

- **Compromising:**   Let's see what we can agree on
                                and then split the difference

- **Collaborating:**   Win:Win dynamics and a search for
                                mutually beneficial outcomes

- **Avoiding:**   Moving away either to prevent further
                                loss and damage or as a strategy

- **Accommodating:**   OK, let's see what we can do, and
                                let's keep it friendly OK?

Fig. 8.16   Five conflict management styles.

may prefer to use some and perhaps opt out of, or dismiss as unhelpful, those remaining. Each though has its role and the more flexible you can be in responding to conflict and challenge the more able you will be to maintain productive work relationships and meet some, if not all, of your objectives. The disadvantage of only relying on one or two of these styles is that you could use them in inappropriate situations. This will reduce your effectiveness and well-being.

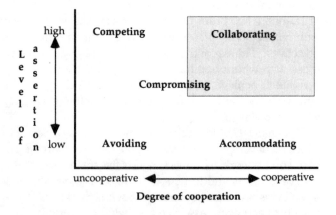

Fig. 8.17   A model of conflict management (Thomas, 1976).

Figure 8.17 shows the styles in relation to the degree of assertiveness and cooperation they utilize. In thinking about Fig. 8.17 and the definitions of the five styles, think back on how you seem to work through conflict situations with colleagues, patients, relatives, friends etc. Try to guess where you would place yourself in the figure to reflect the ways you generally work. You may like to think of others and see if this diagram gives a clue about how they seem, from your experience of them, to tackle conflict.

The lightly shaded area indicates an area where both the level of assertion and the degree of cooperation is high. It is likely that if you are able to combine these features in your efforts to resolve problems you will feel more positive about what you have been trying to achieve and the way in which you have gone about it. Working in a collaborative way allows more scope for each party to achieve some of their aims and sets the scene for a more constructive way of working together in the future.

If this makes sense to you, you could use these ideas as part of your preparation for forthcoming situations where you anticipate there will be some differences of opinion. You can remind yourself of the five styles and then decide the optimum one(s) to use.

Take a look at Fig. 8.18. How often do you use these ways of resolving – or at least getting through – conflict situations? Completing Fig. 8.18 may help you realize how often, or how infrequently, you make use of all five strategies. Make no mistake, although 'collaborating' is of considerable value there are times when the other styles are better.

	Rarely	Occasionally	Regularly	A lot	Always
Competing					
Compromising					
Collaborating					
Avoiding					
Accommodating					

Fig. 8.18 My use of the conflict management styles.

You may also want to select two colleagues, one whom you see as very successful in handling situations of conflict and negotiation, and one who does not have those skills. You could record the extent to which they use these styles and see what profiles emerge. This could give a clue as to what underlies their operational success, or lack of it!

From your responses it may become clear to you that you tend to rely on some of these styles more than others. Some may be neglected or not used by you at all. If this is the case you may be less successful than you could be in handling conflicts. You may wish to consider extending your range of approach to give you more flexibility for the future through, skills training, coaching on-the-job by colleagues and practice.

If you have identified that you rely heavily on only one or two of these options it is very likely that you will have behaved inappropriately in some cases. Perhaps one of the styles you did not use would have been more constructive. You may also be prone to misdiagnose situations to 'fit' the type of responses you feel more comfortable with rather than to the conflict situation to which you have to respond. It is like that old saying that if the only tool you have is a hammer you will see everything that comes along as something to hit!

There are other resolution outcomes that are rewarding other than solely winning. One of the problems with working to win each time is that there will be losers. They will probably store up resentments and look for ways to get their own back and to beat you next time. A powerful way of intervening in a dispute or a conflict situation is to see if there are any ways in which a win–lose scenario could be shifted to become a win–win one, where each party is able to gain or secure something they value from the situation.

One of the most dangerous outcomes of a total 'win' is the deep sense of loss and humiliation that the loser(s) may feel. If this happens, they are likely to be preoccupied with getting their own back. Not only can this be of overriding importance to them but you may have to divert energy and attention to protecting yourself from them as soon as you become aware of what is going to happen.

This can lead to major strife and reduce the effectiveness of the ward or clinic. It can also disrupt the delivery of care. It is very easy to under-estimate the power and intensity of staff who feel they have 'lost out', been 'wronged' or in some way not been treated fairly. This sense of injustice can go back many years but can be 'reactivated' in the present as if it had only happened yesterday. Here again is the importance of finding out about the history of the relationship because it does influence current relationships and the definition of the current issues to be resolved.

On the ward, and in working with colleagues, you may like to think about *how* you instruct colleagues to do the work you have directed them to do. Review how you talk and relate to patients, especially if you perceive them to be difficult, which is often shorthand for saying: they won't immediately do what you asked them to. It may be that, inad-vertently, you are storing up trouble for yourself in the future. This is especially so if you notice that you are too keen on trying to win when you could also adopt more collaborative options.

Don't forget:

- that it is often easier to disagree than agree,
- how we often look for difficulties and faults,

- the impact of the organization's culture on management style,
- to separate the people from the issues in a conflict,
- to explore each party's interests rather than jump to solutions.

Bullying and intimidation at work

Harassment and bullying at work are increasingly being recognized as major problem areas that demand more attention and control. While sexual harassment has been an area of attention for several years, after decades of neglect, it is only in the last couple of years that bullying and harassment have emerged into the spotlight.

Being bullied and harassed has a devastating and long-standing impact on our psychological, and possibly physical, well-being. We may well have disturbing memories related to some aspect of bullying, of being bullied, of bullying others, or of watching others being bullied. If we were bullied we may think that it was in fact our fault and that, in some way, we actually invited this behaviour. That, for example, we should have stood up for ourselves more effectively, or that we really should have been better at our work. We may have memories of being taunted and ridiculed publicly, or memories perhaps of how we showed ourselves unable to fight back.

What about if, on reading this, you realize *you* were a bully to other people and that you operated in ways that caused extreme distress to others through your treatment of them. How do you feel about that now? Pleasure, remorse, or that it was a long time ago and is best forgotten?

What if we all have within us the potential to be the bully and the person who could be bullied. If this is so, what is it that decides which way we will go? What would cause us to shift to the alternative position? Is there a chain reaction where we are bullied by one person and in turn we then bully someone else? If this is so, how do you stop the chain reaction?

There was a very popular TV series many years ago in which one of the main catch phrases was '. . . I didn't get where I was today by . . .' It suggests that we are influenced in our present behaviour by past experiences, by what we have seen or been told we have to do to get on and be successful. Demonstrating your competence by imposing your view over another's contains elements of a bullying approach. While not inducing us at all to be bullies, these ways nevertheless encourage an almost aggressive presentation of oneself to succeed. In one's desire to do well, it may be that this can encourage you to adopt a pushy, bullying way of working with others which, if successful, is likely to be retained. You could say, it works – and anyway people should stand up for themselves.

The trouble however is that bullying will often take place without witnesses, or only when there are others present who too are involved in the bullying process. It can also be presented as a 'right of passage' –

that a person *has* to endure some degree of harassment. That to object, speak out about, or 'blow the whistle' would indicate that person's non-suitability and inability to be able to take on the job or role. A web of complicity and a pseudo-rationalization for bullying and intimidation at work can be created which makes it even harder for the bullied to resist, be listened to and tell others.

It is also organizationally embarrassing and distasteful for a senior manager or director to accept that within their organization such practices could be going on. Where at all possible, it is likely that they will prefer such matters to be pushed under the carpet and informally stopped. This, however, does not help the bullied person (or group) who, by raising their concerns, have made themselves very vulnerable by speaking out. They could make themselves vulnerable to further attack, professional scrutiny and pressure to leave or to retract their accusations. What can you do if the potential for bullying at work exists, but where it is very difficult to get others to listen and examine your claims? There seem to me to be several things you can do. They all revolve around collecting information and building up your case at the professional, institutional and personal level as shown in Fig. 8.19.

	Your Experience	Do this.....	Action to take	Focus
Professional	intimidation during training	collect evidence get corroboration	confront, backed by data	address the issue
Organisational				
	management style, org style	ditto	ditto	ditto
Personal	bullying	reality test your experience	confront and assert yourself	re-definition of the relationship

Fig. 8.19 Strategic responses to bullying at work.

The critical actions are to collect evidence of what is going on, and to build up information that can be confirmed by others. Advice, support and guidance from your professional body – as long as it is confidential at this stage – is likely to prove both reassuring and prudent. If there is confidential staff support or an occupational health service, they could also be involved at some stage.

One means through which, in spite of being bullied or intimidated, you can become more able and prepared to resist will be if you have a stronger belief in yourself and what you stand for. You can then be more prepared to raise these matters and have them looked at, as well as having more confidence in your daily work. So being positive about yourself, your accomplishments, your values and beliefs is a necessary prerequisite to resist bullying and harassment.

In addition, you will need to assess the evidence you have collected objectively and dispassionately to see how it would look to a neutral third party. Finally, you will need to assert your views and experience of bullying and be prepared to stand your ground when challenged. In short, you will need to present influentially and effectively. To do this you may need to use a model as a basis for your approach.

Influencing behaviours and strategies

What follows are some ideas about effective influence. They work and are simple to remember. They are not always put into practice because most of us have been taught that the way to influence others is to force our point of view on the other person. The approach outlined in Fig. 8.20 doesn't work like that.

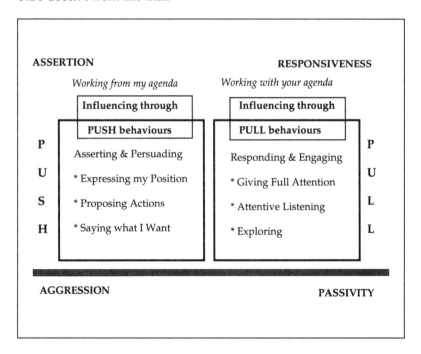

Fig. 8.20 A model for personal influence (positive and constructive behaviours to adopt).

The following approach suggests that there are two main ways in which you can work more effectively with others and exercise *positive* influence.

Firstly, be clear about what you want, and then back it up with logic and reason. *Secondly*, listen fully and with respect to their point of view so that you understand their position and can then begin to work *with* them in a more informed way.

A push–pull model for effective influence

The approach uses a mix of assertive (push) and responsive (pull) behaviour as shown in Fig. 8.20. It is the combination of both push and pull behaviour that will increase your ability to work with others and improve your influence rather than relying on just pushing for what you want.

The figure presents a model of influence, where the emphasis is on being assertive. At the same time the emphasis is on being genuinely open and responsive to the needs of those you are trying to influence. On the left-hand side of the model are the three assertive behaviours which present your case and the outcomes you want to secure. Here the emphasis is on assertively pushing for what you want working from *your agenda*.

On the right-hand side the emphasis is on attending to the views and stance of the other person. Your aim here is to understand, as fully as you can, how they see things and what they want. Here you are engaging with them and responding by giving them considerable attention. This is about engaging with them and working with *their agenda*.

These two ways of working operate together to give you a way of structuring your work with others. Below the solid line is the dysfunctional behaviour of *passivity*, which is what happens if I am too responsive to your needs. *Aggression* is another dysfunctional behaviour which is what happens if I go too far in pushing for what I want and try to beat you down.

The 'push' behaviours – asserting and persuading

On the left side are the *push behaviours* and it is through using these that you demonstrate to others

- what you want
- the action steps needed
- why it is important to you
- the facts, logic and reason of your position.

The underlying purpose of your behaviour is to push them towards agreeing with your proposals, ideas and intentions. The whole thrust of this side of the model is about *pushing* for what you want to achieve, backed up by facts and reason. You are working from what you seek to achieve from *your agenda*. You are quite clear about that by saying exactly what you *want* (something, incidentally, which many people find extremely difficult to do). If this is a difficulty for you, it can help by saying '... I want ...' to yourself out loud. This may sound a little strange but, perhaps surprisingly, it will help you to use the phrase more readily with someone else.

Use the following sequence to help you build up your case step-by-step in a way that does not threaten or violate the other person:

(1) *Expressing my position:* you let the other person know where you stand in relation to the issue and why, drawing on relevant information, facts and figures, etc.

(2) *Proposing actions:* building on from (1) you can now introduce proposals for what you consider appropriate to do, which are realistic and viable given the information available.

(3) *Saying what I want:* if the intended outcome has not yet occurred, you state firmly and assertively, but not aggressively or in a threatening way, what you want. This will already have been based on your analysis of the situation given the information available to you.

(4) *Repeating and reasserting:* sometimes it is necessary to reassert the sequence (1)–(3) together. This has the effect of showing your well-thought-out proposition and your clarity of reasoned purpose.

Of course, following this sequence is no guarantee that you will be successful in achieving your objectives. However, it offers you a pattern and a procedure to follow that is coherent, that slowly builds up your case and gets you to say what you *want* from the other person or that situation. It is likely to be far more influential than not having your position clear in your mind. By clarifying what you want, you will not need to rely on the emotional force of your proposition to carry the day.

On its own though, it is not sufficient to build positive working relationships. You may be able to achieve your objectives but, if you relied on this way of influence all the time, you may not generate collaborative working relationships with many people. All they would consider is that you get your way most of the time and that you seem to have little interest in them. So, the 'push' needs to be balanced by attending to, and understanding, what your colleagues need and how they see things from their point of view. This is where the right side of the model comes into play.

The 'pull' behaviours – responding and engaging

The essence of the right side is that you seek to understand and engage with the other person on the issues and perspectives as they see them. In other words you work with them on *their agenda*, not yours. This means listening very carefully and attentively to their views and perspectives. You must put your wants and wishes temporarily into the background to appreciate the other person's view.

Through working in this way you can begin to see if there are areas of joint agreement, where and why the differences between you exist and if there are any ways in which the differences could be bridged. This is the *pull* side of the model and it balances the push side.

One feature of this side of the model is that it builds up rapport and mutual appreciation if it is done well. This is because you are concentrating on the other person rather than continuing to push only for your preferred point of view.

There is a sequence to follow here also:

(1) *Giving full attention:* here you focus on the other person and their situation. You deliberately put your own issues and objectives into the background.
(1) *Attentive listening:* this is one of the most influential behaviours where you work solely from the material they give you, both facts and feelings, and demonstrate through reflecting back and interpreting that you do indeed understand their position.
(3) *Exploring:* because of (1) and (2) you are able to explore their material more fully with sensitivity and care, and build greater mutual understanding, although not necessarily agreement.

The format of this model is simple. You need to know what you want to achieve and you should be able to back this up in ways that are understandable to others. You should be prepared to say what you want in a firm manner. At the same time you need to be open to the views of others and genuinely willing to listen fully and with respect. Thus you will be able to appreciate their position as fully as possible.

It is through combining these complementary strategies that you create a balanced influencing approach that emphasizes your responsiveness and sensitivity to the needs of the other person. At the same time you can define what you are seeking to achieve. You rely neither on pushing for what you want nor on being totally responsive to the needs of others as a means of influence. It is the mix of the two that makes the difference.

While it is productive and constructive to be able to stand up for yourself and push for what you want, it can become counter-productive if you are preoccupied with your own needs to the exclusion of others. This can lead you to be seen and experienced as an *aggressive*, rather than as an assertive, person whose priority is to impose their needs on others.

Similarly, it is very constructive to be responsive to the needs of others and to understand their position fully. Yet here also there are dangers to watch out for. If you become too responsive to the needs of the other person you could find that you lose sight of your own needs. The danger here is of *passivity*. You become like a piece of putty unable to maintain your shape and integrity in dealing with others.

In Fig. 8.21 the positive and productive influencing behaviours (above the horizontal line) are contrasted with those that are not productive or constructive (below the line).

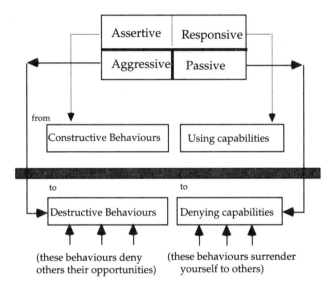

Fig. 8.21   Contrasting positive and negative influencing behaviour.

Assertion is about expressing your wants in a firm way. This needs to be achieved in a manner that in no way demeans or threatens the person to whom you are speaking, or denies them their rights either. It is about stating what you want firmly even when challenged, but not by resorting to aggression or negative behaviour.

To do this you need to be clear about what and why; what you are after is important to you and you need to feel good and positive about yourself too. Being assertive is not about bluster and blurting out loudly and emotionally what you want. It is an altogether more focused, calmly executed affair and practised way of working. A large part of your effectiveness in influencing others is in how they see you and how you come across to them.

The 'words', the 'music' and the 'dance'

Although assertiveness is a way of stating what you want, this is only a part of the procedure. It is also important *how* you communicate, to be more specific: how you use your body to communicate. Much of what we are influenced by comes from what we see in front of us. In being assertive a great deal of your resolve will show itself in how you physically manage your stance, your posture and the gestures you use. All of this will be noticed, and watched for, by the person with whom you are interacting. Of course, the words you use matter; there has to be sufficient sense there for people to believe enough in what is being said. However, body stance, posture and movement, exercise a significant influence on the overall impact you make. In many ways, we are what our behaviour suggests we are.

The impact of any message you seek to convey is made up or three main components which are

- *what* you say,
- *how* you say it and the,
- *use of the body* during the communication.

You need to pay attention to the *words*, the *music* and the *dance* (which refers to your body movements).

From your experience what do you think would be the most and the least influential of these three? For example, if you think about the impact of a communication with others how would you distribute this impact in terms of these three components? Do it yourself first by using Fig. 8.22 below. Then you can ask colleagues to do the same and plot their responses for subsequent discussion.

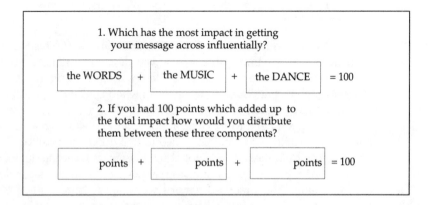

Fig. 8.22   Where does the impact come from?

If you were able to get some suggestions from colleagues, there were probably some large differences between the emphasis that was placed on these three features of communication. It is likely that the *words* scored quite highly. After all in our training and education a great deal of emphasis is placed on this component; on putting together a logical argument. Also in marshalling the facts and giving a report that is understandable and clear.

Some attention is given to introducing variation in how we say things to add life and interest to the words being used. This is about the pitch, rhythm, power, speed and the pauses, as well as emphasis you give to what you say. So, the *music* is something you may have been told to consider at some time but probably with the emphasis remaining on the logic of the argument to be presented as the primary focus for attention.

The *dance* is all about how you present yourself physically and how you use your body during a communication. This covers how you stand, sit and move around, the gestures you use and if you fidget. It is about your use of space, eye contact and touch as well as expressions, facial movements and posture.

You will be most influential when all three components are in tune with each other. You will then be able to present in a coherent and congruent manner. The message you express will be articulated with pace, pause and interest, and this will be perfectly in tune with the gestures, movements and posture used during your communication.

Some studies have been done into the relative importance of the words, music and the dance in influencing the impact of the communication on recipients. This suggests that of the three it is the dance which is the most influential. It is suggested that the gestures, posture, the physical 'presence' we bring to our communications exercise a major influence on how others respond to what we say. While it is necessary to have a believable proposition to make, it will probably not be the message itself (the words) that will decide if people act on what we say, but how we say it backed up by the dance.

Of the three, only about 10% of the impact comes from the words, about 35% from the music with the remaining 55% from the dance. These percentages should be taken as an indication of relative impact. Do not get fixed on the precise figures but look at the overall message that these figures suggest. They suggest that how we present and how we manage our physical impact is very significant in influencing others. It has far more impact than a perfectly crafted and beautifully worded presentation on its own. It would seem that while we may admire the eloquent argument we are unlikely to accept it unless it is presented with impact and belief.

This is in sharp contrast to most of the training received by professionals where the overwhelming emphasis is on hard data and facts. In addition to being clear about the facts, etc., these findings suggest that coaching and feedback sessions about our behaviour could significantly enhance our influencing effectiveness.

If you apply this to your own experience does it appear valid? Think about those around you who are influential. What are they saying, how do they say it and how do they present themselves in their work with others? It may be worth seeing how much emphasis you give to the words, music and the dance. When you are working with others watch and note what they actually *do*, and try to see what effect this has on their ability to work and influence you.

Concluding comments

This chapter has emphasized the inherent difficulty in working with others and introduced several models and frameworks. You can use these to diagnose what is happening in a situation and then take action from a more informed position. Disagreements will occur, differences exist. The question is not how to make us all agree and become the same, but how to acknowledge and work with the differences and difficulties in productive and ethical ways.

Reference

Thomas, K. (1976) Conflict and conflict management in *Handbook of Industrial and Organizational Psychology* M. Dunnette (ed), Rand McNally, Skokie, IL.

Further reading

Adams, A. (1992) *Bullying at Work*, Virago Press, London.

Berbe, E. (1964) *Games People Play*, Penguin Books, Harmondsworth.

Fisher, R. and Ury, W. (1983) *Getting to Yes*, Penguin Books, Harmondsworth.

Hamilton, J. and Kiefer, M. (1986) *Survival Skills For the New Nurse*, JB Lippincott, Philadelphia.

Hase, S. and Douglas, A. (1986) *Human Dynamics and Nursing*, Churchill Livingstone, Edinburgh.

Honey, P. (1992) *Problem People . . . and How to Manage Them*, Institute of Personnel Management, London.

Horne, E. and Cowan, T. (1992) *Effective Communication: Some Nursing Perspectives*, Wolfe Publishing Co, London.

Jongeward, D. and James, M. (1981) *Winning Ways in Health Care*, Addison-Wesley, Reading, Ma.

Kennedy, E. (1975) *If You Really Knew Me, Would You Still Like Me?* Argus Communications, Niles, IL.

King, N. (1987) *The First Five Minutes*, Simon and Schuster, London.

Luft, J. (1963) *Group Processes*, The National Press, Palo Alto.

Masson, J. (1988) *Against Therapy*, Fontana London.

McKenna, E. (1994) *Business Psychology and Organisational Behaviour*, Lawrence Erlbaum Associates, Hove.

Nelson-Jones, R. (1993) *You Can Help!*, Cassell, London.

O'Leary, J., Wendelgass, S. and Zimmerman, H. (1986) *Winning Strategies for Nursing Managers*, JB Lippincott, Philadelphia.

Priestly, P. *et al.* (1978) *Social Skills and Personal Problem Solving*, Tavistock Publications, London.

Rutter, P. (1990) *Sex in the Forbidden Zone*, Unwin Hyman, London.

Spinelli, E. (1994) *Demystifying Therapy*, Constable, London.

Chapter 9
Meetings, Groups and Teams

Introduction

The next two chapters look at what happens when people work in groups, either as part of a specified team or in a more general meeting. I have used these terms rather flexibly in these chapters because they are all different types of collective work groupings, which is where the focus of the chapters lies. I didn't want to become too bogged down in having to define the differences between them all the time. Take it as given that the discussion and points raised will apply generally, even if only one of the terms e.g. team, is used in the text.

This chapter introduces a six 'R' framework for looking at groups, teams and meetings. You can use it to review a group's effectiveness, for the setting up of a group, to plan for effective meetings or to guide team performance. Chapter 10 puts particular emphasis on the dynamics, roles and interactions that make people in groups so interesting, unpredictable and, at times, so difficult to be part of.

There is a great deal written about groups, meetings and teams because they are an inescapable part of our life. Whether they are formally constituted like a committee, or informal 'off-the-record' chats between three or four people, the dynamics that arise when people get together significantly affect individual behaviour both positively and negatively, also the development of ideas, the taking of decisions, self-esteem, motivation, etc.

I expect you can recall how you have felt elated, well regarded, and determined to do well after some meetings. Other times it was quite the opposite. You ended up feeling dispirited, frustrated, devalued and depressed. No doubt there were teams and groups you were delighted to be associated with, and part of. There may have been others where you did your best to disguise your membership, or where in some way it was so unpleasant, you couldn't wait to move on elsewhere.

These chapters will help you to look at some of the things that go on in meetings, teams and groups so that in the future you will be able to begin to unpick some of the underlying processes that occur. If you are able to look more closely at what is happening you will then have more of an opportunity to intervene constructively. Thus you will be able to influence the course of events. At the very least, you will become more able to represent the interests you are responsible for covering and look after your own personal interests as well.

As you go through these chapters, remember to relate the perspectives I cover to your own experiences and what you recall others telling you about theirs. You already have a tremendous store of experience and knowledge about group behaviour. However, you may not yet have looked at it in an ordered way to find out just how much you do know.

The practical advantage of the material in this chapter is that you will be able to apply it to situations where there are a number of you working together. This could be in a team working on a task that needs to be completed, on the ward round, or it could be during a case conference.

Understanding group behaviour involves noting and making sense of what the members of the group are doing, the type of responses they give to others and so on. The detail is important but so is the overall flow and shape of how the group is functioning. Don't try to catch everything that is going on because you will just be overwhelmed and bogged down by too much detail. Try to balance the detail with the general picture and pattern of working that is developing in the group.

To begin with you may get more insight by keeping your eye on the overall pattern and flow and on the critical dynamics and incidents of the meeting. When you are more confident begin to focus on the more detailed interactions as well. I expect you will always cover some of both of these dimensions so it is a question of where, and when, to put the emphasis.

So, take it easy don't try to capture everything that is happening, try to watch for an overall pattern and track the behaviour and interventions of the key people. As you make more regular use of the ideas that follow you will be able to keep track of more and more dimensions. Looking at groups is fascinating, intriguing, productive and leads to insight about yourself and others. Listen to what you can and use the ideas to see your experiences in a different light. See if you can begin to bring the ideas and perspective outlined into use for yourself wherever you may be.

Before we go any further select a group, a team or a meeting that you are part of and with which you have worked at least three or four times. With that grouping in mind can you complete the following questionnaire in Fig. 9.1? Use the SA (strongly agree) to SD (strongly disagree) rating scale with NS (not sure) as the mid-point for use in emergencies only!

How did your scores come out? Could you look again at your responses to see if there were any underlying themes that strike you as interesting or important to note. For example, is there clarity about purpose, do people have defined roles or is it a bit of a hit-and-miss affair. Do you (and some others) feel that your contributions are wanted

	SA	A	NS	D	SD
1 I know what we are there to do					
2 I am clear what is expected of me					
3 I am allowed to freely contribute					
4 We seem to fight each other					
5 It is very competitive					
6 We get things done					
7 I know who is responsible for team leadership					
8 We know in advance what we've to discuss					
9 Follow up notes confirm what we agreed					
10 I feel encouraged to contribute					
11 A lot seems to be agreed outside the meetings					
12 The meetings drag and go on too long					
13 There are clear roles					
14 There seem to be 'in' and 'out' groupings					
15 Attendance is very poor					
16 People get there on time and generally stay					
17 We manage our time very well					
18 All the agenda items are regularly covered					
19 Items and papers are often tabled at the meeting					
20 I enjoy these meetings					

Fig. 9.1   Health check: 20 questions on meetings/group workings.

and valued, or superfluous and a nuisance. The 20 questions were to start you thinking about these matters before we look at them later in the chapter.

Although for the purposes of these chapters I am going to use the words *groups*, *teams* and *meetings* more or less interchangeably as if there were no differences between them I see:

- *A team* is either a very specific grouping of specified people who have been brought together, on some selected basis, to undertake some defined piece of work. Or it is a regular team of colleagues who work together as their primary work responsibilities in getting specified work completed.

- *A group* could be used synonymously with team but it could also refer to a grouping of people who are less clearly related. They still have some specified, but looser, working association which draws them together from time to time.
- *A meeting* can comprise people from dissimilar groups and organizations who are drawn together for that meeting(s) or who are drawn from a larger team of existing group for a particular specified purpose.

Two considerations of overriding importance each and every time a group of people meet are *what* are we here to do and *how* are we going to accomplish the work we have met to do?

These are so central to everything that occurs in groups of people that it is amazing just how frequently one – or both – are not made clear or raised in discussion. Failure to do this (leading to groups losing their sense of focus and purpose etc.) could be one of the main reasons meetings are viewed by so many participants as inefficient, ineffective and 'a waste of time'. Perhaps it is because they seem so obvious and self-apparent that they are often neglected. It is as if each person assumed the others were clear and were agreed about these two pivotal questions. You will recall from the last chapter however, that this is not the case at all.

It seems to me that there is a great deal that can be done to improve the performance and productivity of groups, teams and meetings. Primarily this is by clarifying their purpose and maintaining a focus on what (and how) the objectives are to be achieved.

Your experiences though may be different to mine and I would like you to draw on yours. As a start think back to meetings you have been involved in. Make a note of two or three very productive ones and two or three where it seemed to you that very little was achieved and where, frankly, they were awful. Now can you be specific about what went on? You may want to focus only on one of the positive experiences and one of the unproductive meetings to start with. What was it which seemed to help or hinder effective group workings? Don't worry if your recollections come out all jumbled – just make a note of your thoughts. Finally, working from your notes speculate about what caused the problems in those meetings and what made things go well recording your thoughts on Fig. 9.2.

I would like you to refer back to these notes as you work through the chapter. There may be additional insights and perspectives that you will want to add to these initial notes as we progress. At the same time I hope you will use the material to reconsider what may be going on in the meetings you go to and in the work groups of which you are currently a part.

The rest of this chapter sets out a six-dimensional framework to look

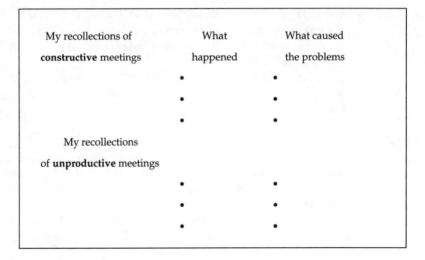

My recollections of **constructive** meetings	What happened	What caused the problems
•		•
•		•
•		•
My recollections of **unproductive** meetings		
•		•
•		•
•		•

Fig. 9.2   Recollections of productive and unproductive meetings.

at any group, team or meeting that you are involved with to see more clearly what it is doing and how productive it appears to be.

A six 'R' framework for looking at groups, teams and meetings

This is a framework to help you to structure and focus your attention onto six key dimensions of group working. The dimensions are shown in Fig. 9.3.

The key to effective performance is shared clarity of purpose. You will recall from Chapter 3 how this was shown to be at the heart of things in the Galbraith model of organization. It is the same with groups, teams and in meetings. I continue to be amazed how often a meeting lurches into action, often without an agenda and often with the participants not fully clear on what they are there to do. I've shown the 'work' to be done at the centre point of Fig. 9.4.

The six areas shown in Fig. 9.4 need to be looked at and worked through if the team, group or meeting is to function in a focused, productive and mutually rewarding way. There will always be differences of opinion and belief. There will invariably be errors and mistakes made. In hindsight we will sometimes realize that we should have made a different decision and that our diagnosis of the situation was in some respects inaccurate or inadequate. However, if you are able to look carefully at these six dimensions, and work through them with those involved, you will reduce many of the current frustrations experienced in working teams, groups and in meetings.

1. the **WORK REQUIREMENTS** to be done, the purpose for the group

2. the **ROLES**, both formal and informal, to be taken

3. the **RULES** and procedures to be followed

4. the types of **RELATIONSHIPS** encouraged (and discouraged)

5. the culture and tone, the mutual **RESPECT & REGARD** in the group

Through attending to these dimensions the hope would be that as an effective and productive group

6. the **RESULTS** needed would be achieved and in ways that

enhanced individual and group working relationships and morale

Fig. 9.3 The six 'R' framework in outline.

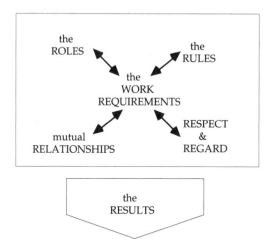

Fig. 9.4 Clarifying the purpose: what are we here to do?

These aspects of group working do not reflect the whole story because there will be other, personal differences, interactional dimensions, historical features and unconscious influences that inject more complexity into the situation. Yet attending to these six dimensions will improve individual and group satisfaction and performance.

1. The work requirements

Of all the dimensions this one is fundamental. If there is no valid purpose or specific work to do then there is no need for the group, team or the meeting! You need to determine:

- What is the purpose for the meeting?
- What sort of contributions will be called for?
- Is it a meeting
    - to decide something
    - to discuss possibilities
    - to build more shared understandings about a topic or issue
    - a planning meeting, or
    - a meeting for those present to be given more information and news?
- Does the meeting have some symbolic purpose?
- Is it to sanction or give approval to some work others have now completed?

Each of these differing purposes reflect the type of work to be covered. If things are to go as constructively as they can, this will be understood and appreciated by those who are present.

Serious disruptive behaviour can result if there is a big mismatch between what people thought the meeting was for and what transpires.

Think back to more meetings you have been in where things really did go well. Then think of other examples where the meeting was appalling; where it didn't go well at all. Use the questions below to note your recollections adding in where you think the problems occurred:

- Was I clear about the purpose of the meeting?
- Did I know what was expected of me before the meeting, during the meeting or after the meeting?
- Did the setting and facilities, numbers and materials, agenda, papers etc., match the purpose stated?

How would you describe the scenarios in Fig. 9.5 and what would you expect to be the consequences for the person talking about them?

These have come from my experiences. I have my view about what was going on in each and what needed to be changed, if anything, to make it better next time. Have you had similar experiences to mine? Perhaps you could make a note of four or five recent meetings:

(1) Briefly describe what happened.
(2) Note how you felt about what went on.
(3) What were the contributions you made?

(4)   What impact did you make?

(5)   What you would like to be different, if anything, next time?

S1: 'I come to this meeting full of ideas and we got talked at for ninety minutes flat. Then the boss left!'

S2: 'I don't know what they expect, we were asked to suggest ways of improving savings; I talked about time scheduling and better hand over meetings – the rest wanted to talk about supply and ordering procedures'.

S3: 'It was great. We all had the papers to look at in advance and reach our initial solution – so we talked it out and agreed what to go for.'

S4: 'We certainly aired the issues – about three times – but it took ages to move beyond these circular discussions and we never did decide before we ran out of time, that seems to happen a lot recently!

Fig. 9.5   Comments from four meetings.

	Meeting A	Meeting B	Meeting C	Meeting D
(i) what happened				
(ii) my feelings about the meeting				
(iii) my contributions				
(iv) the impact they had				
(iv) what could be better next time				

Fig. 9.6   Reviewing some of my recent meetings.

At the end of this chapter, you will be able to review these recollections and be clearer about what you could do, or encourage others to do, to remedy any shortfalls you may have identified.

Reviewing meetings by jotting down your impressions of what went on, or working it through in your head, is a very productive habit. It ensures you habitually consciously reflect on your experiences and begin to consider what changes, if any, may be needed next time. Another very good habit is to validate your perceptions with a couple of colleagues who were also present. This way you will get a more rounded picture and assessment. But keep it quick and simple, and get into this 'review and reflection' habit.

By doing this 'snappy' type of review you can be alerted to the ways of working that you habitually use. There is nothing wrong with this unless they are unproductive. Also these quick reviews will alert you to the types of roles or situations you find yourself moving into in groups and meetings. Once again if you find these appealing and productive, all well and good. If however you are not happy with them, you may want to think about how to reduce this happening, or to stop it altogether in the future.

Clarifying the purpose of the meeting is important. If it is not made clear to every attendee you have a recipe for disharmony, wasted time and frustration. If you are running the meeting, be clear why it is needed, what has to be done and what the outcome must be. If, for example, the meeting is to review the ward situation without any specific tasks to be completed, confirm that a free and open discussion is the objective for this meeting. Openly reconfirming the purpose reassures those present and emphasises what is expected of the participants.

In each meeting there may be several different purposes depending on the items on the agenda. You may find it very helpful to indicate against each agenda item what is wanted, as illustrated in Fig. 9.7.

Guard against confusion of purpose. Wherever possible the work to be done, especially for a project group, should be set out in either a project brief or in formalized terms of reference. This is a critical document because it is the touchstone for decisions about who should be involved. It also refers to what skills are needed, the frequency of meetings and the performance criteria seen as relevant to assess progress and performance etc.

I did some research several years ago that looked at the committee structure in a health authority. Almost all of the committees I monitored and researched had no formal terms of reference. Not surprisingly they were very unhappy when this fact emerged. It exposed these groups as not being at all clear about what they were there to do. I also found most of them to be unproductive talk-shops where the status of membership of this or that committee seemed to me to be more important than resolving business issues. Most of the actual decision making seemed to be made by the key players outside the formal committees. The role of the formal committees was then often relegated to rubber stamping these informal, out of committee, discussions.

A g e n d a:

1. Review of bed state, current and projected (for discussion)

2. Allocation of discretionary monies (to decide on appropriate action)

3. Minutes of Trust Board meeting(to receive for information)

4. Request for procedures review from Clinical Director
   (to agree next steps)

5. Update from clinical Business Manager (discussion & review)

Etc. etc.

Fig. 9.7 Ward review meeting: Saracen ward – 15.5.95.

Having a clear remit is vital for sharpening performance and using members' skills and experience. Members of groups, teams and meetings will then know more clearly how they fit in and value and enjoy their contribution.

2. The roles, both formal and informal

Depending on the purpose and the outcomes wanted there are various roles within the group, and in a meeting, that need to be covered to facilitate completion of the work. This can be done in several different ways. Much depends on the nature of the work to be done and the culture of the department or unit. It often surprises me to see, in different places, how groups have set up different ways of organizing themselves to do the same, or very similar, work. These differences reflect the local organization's culture and the different work settings. As you have moved around the service you must have experienced this too.

Roles such as chairperson, recorder of decisions etc., can be:

- formally designated,
- informally assigned, or
- they can be encouraged to evolve as the group begins to work together and find its feet.

Often the professional and organizational hierarchy will determine who will take the lead and be responsible for a group's work based on seniority. This is not always the best option unless the work to be done is within that person's expertise. If it is not, it may put them under unnecessary pressure to demonstrate a competence they don't possess. They may be tempted to try to bluff their way through so as not to lose face or to somehow 'prove' themselves.

A better option is to decide who needs to be involved. This can be based on the mix of skills, experience and stature required to complete the work successfully. Putting to one side the seniority of the people involved consider who could best occupy the key formal and informal roles to be covered. Finally, put the seniority and professional issues back in place to finalize how that group can realistically function.

Roles in meetings and groups can be fixed and determined in advance or they can be covered to allow several people in turn to undertake them. Sometimes there is a deliberate policy to change the chairperson regularly on an agreed basis. This can be done for internal political reasons as well as for personal development ones.

Bear in mind that I am talking here of multidisciplinary groups and meetings that are outside the formal reporting hierarchy where I would anticipate those meetings and work groups to be usually chaired by the most senior person present, although here again they may not be the best person to undertake that responsibility. It does seem a great shame that there is a general assumption that the most senior graded person should take the chair. It is perfectly feasible to retain one's senior position – and indeed enhance one's professional standing – by allowing those more junior to you to take the lead, where appropriate, with your support and sanction.

What sort of roles need to be covered? There are a set of roles that are primarily concerned to 'make it happen' (*task achievement roles*). There are also roles that will 'help' the group work more effectively together (group effectiveness or *'facilitative' roles*). Both are vitally important. While the facilitative roles may, on occasion, be formally designated they are more often taken on informally and shared between the members. There are some dangers and problems associated in formally designating facilitative roles, in that to do so:

- can feel a bit false,
- suggests that those who don't have such a role designed to them have a reduced responsibility to help the group work well together,
- can set up some resistance to those with a facilitative brief from those who don't,
- can offend those not given a facilitative role as most people like to feel they have skills in these areas.

The important thing to remember is that both sets of roles need to be covered during meetings and within teams. Some examples of the types of roles are set out in Fig. 9.8.

'Making it happen' roles	Facilitative roles
# setting targets	# diagnosing group processes
# providing relevant data	# summarising differences
# proposing solutions	# clarifying
# defining resources	# bringing in non-contributors
# specifying constraints	# de-fusing tension
# pushing for decisions	

Fig. 9.8 Some task achievement and facilitative roles.

Several writers and researchers have identified specific roles, derived from their research and from watching groups in action, in to what makes for effective teams (see Chapter 10). But for the moment stay with this fundamental distinction between roles and behaviours intended to help the work get done, and those that help the group or meeting function through attending to the more interactional dynamics taking place.

3. The rules and procedures to follow

If we know what has to be accomplished and have sorted out the roles for this to happen, we then need to discuss the 'rules of engagement'. These will condition our behaviour together and give a framework for our activities. For example, we need to consider such matters as:

- how we will make decisions
- how differences will be resolved
- what we wish to be known for
- how roles and responsibilities will be assigned
- how we will handle conflict
- how we will treat each other
- if we can be honest with each other.

What other 'rules' would you want to be specified in addition to the items noted above?

- ·
- ·
- ·

Matters such as these determine if we will feel able to work confidently with colleagues. I have rarely though found them openly considered. Irrespective of the current task, you need to have agreed professional understandings about these matters. For example that you will work collaboratively with and for each other. That you need to have mutual regard, trust and psychological security knowing that you each have mutual support. This does not mean there won't be difficulties, differences of opinion and practice, but you will know that you are all on the same side.

These understandings are often reflected in the unspoken ways we do things with colleagues. They tend to develop as time passes, but unless some of these ground rules are made explicit, unnecessary worry and tension can be generated and this will impede the speedy integration of people into your teams. Also making explicit the bases from which you need to work together reiterates and reinforces these important aspects of group life and keeps them alive.

If you reflect about the meetings you attend (and the groups you are a part of) what are the rules you notice? Consider both the formally stated ones and those that are followed but not made explicit. Jot them all down (see Fig. 9.9) because they will help you to see more clearly how that meeting (or that group) is organized and how it structures its way of working.

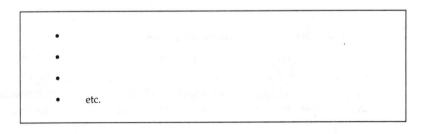

Fig. 9.9   Identifying the formal and informal rules and protocols in use.

If you note the rules and guidelines that are already in use you can identify where more clarity is needed. There may be issues that need to be discussed openly that so far have been neglected or glossed over. Confirming your understanding about the unwritten rules and guidelines that are being followed is a very influential intervention because it brings to the surface some of the hidden ways that the group has been using to order and control itself.

What about your work group? What are the 'rules of engagement' you follow in your work relationships? Do they form a framework that structures and organizes your interactions? Please make a note of what comes to mind in Fig 9.10.

- •
- •
- •
- •   etc.

Fig. 9.10   Group/team rules and protocols we follow.

Such rules put into place a commonly understood framework for your work which colleagues will then expect and can acknowledge as valid. They provide a degree of certainty and that can generate more calmness and predictability about the conduct to be expected from each other. On the other hand, they can lose their positive attributes, and become dysfunctional:

- if they are applied in ways that lose touch with the immediate issues to be addressed,
- when they take on the mantle of ritual and rules for the sake of it (bureaucracy),
- when they make the work even more difficult to complete,
- when they violate people and impede effective work relationships being formed and developed.

In Fig. 9.11 are some examples of 'rules of engagement'. Are they similar to the ones you noted above or have experienced in the past?

Some of the most constructive work any group can do is to spend some time thinking about how they would prefer to work together. Then they need to build up their own framework of guidelines to fit the needs and preferences identified. This will help bind that group together more strongly. They are then likely to value, understand and support each other better at work.

In health care settings this quality of mutual support, value and understanding is especially valuable because of the high pressure and the emotional strain on the nurse. This is important for all staff, not just for nurses. Medical staff, support staff, other professional carers, managerial and administrative staff too need to be aware of these factors.

- We don't attack each other
- Listen first, then explore
- The Chair is neutral
- Roles formalized

more P R O D U C T I V E

- No agenda items for decision without back-up paperwork
- We will work for each other
- It is OK to say 'I don't know'
- We will support each other... etc. etc.

- Shoot first, ask later
- The Chair decides
- Don't talk unless asked

less P R O D U C T I V E

- Get it 'right' or else
- Look after yourself, no one else will
- I don't want your thoughts, I want the facts ... etc. etc.

Fig. 9.11   Rules of engagement: some bases for working together.

4. Types of relationships to encourage

By this stage we know what we have to do. There has been some allocation of roles and responsibilities between us, and we have given some attention to how we want to work together. We have also reached some agreements about mutual support, development and learning etc. So far so good. We can now turn to an aspect of working that is not often separated out for attention, yet has the power to make or break groups and to destroy meetings.

Far too little attention is given to building up and sustaining a constructive and positive spirit in groups and meetings. Often people are watching their backs, keeping their heads down or are preoccupied with trying to look good and score points off others. Critically important matters are often not raised because it won't show that person in a positive light. Good ideas are often not followed up because of rivalries, jealousy or apathy. There can be a worry of being badly treated if one challenges proposals made by a more senior colleague even if this is done constructively. If you doubt this, think back to some of your own experiences. Another way is to look back in history books. Think of examples of catastrophes caused when advisors were too frightened to tell their leaders the true situation, or where political rivalries led courtiers to fight each other rather than the common enemy (see Janis's book *Groupthink* (1982) and Dixon's *On the Psychology of Military Incompetence* (1979).

While the picture may not be a universal one, you will probably recall more than one example of each of the dysfunctional behaviours I have noted. You may even have been personally involved in one or other of them. We have experiences where we became jealous of others' success, especially if we felt that their success (project opportunity, course funding, time off, overtime, secondment etc.) was at the expense of ours. But there is a point beyond which feelings of being let down or jealousy turn to vindictiveness and obsession. It is this level of intensity that I believe we should watch out for. It manifests itself in the persistent unhelpful behaviour noted above.

Why does this occur and what leads us to be so negative and unhelpful? Why do we criticize those around us who may be doing better than we are? Is success and accomplishment a limited commodity, so that if I do well there will be less available for you? Or is there a way whereby we can all do as well as we can?

My view is the latter. Success, accomplishment, good ideas, influence, power etc., are not fixed quantities. We *can* do more to encourage people to enhance themselves yet without diminishing our potential or standing. Mind you success of others may keep us more on our toes, and encourage us to keep more up to date and be more able to handle appropriate challenges from others. Possibly challenges such as these are the reason why we can find ourselves being negative, competitive and dismissive of others. It is possible we instinctively interpret any challenge as a threat which prompts a fight–flight (self-survival) response. Thus without realizing it, to begin with, we are negative about others as a defence against our own fears of incompetence.

However, two ways of keeping at bay these drifts into negative behaviour are:

(1) to decide what type of working relationships are wanted (and then decide how to facilitate this happening),
(2) be clear what type of working relationships and ways of working we don't want (and decide how to guard against them taking hold).

You can sketch this out for yourself for a current group or perhaps from a previous one of which you were a part. If you were just setting up that group, what sort of working relationships would you want to encourage (see Fig. 9.12)?

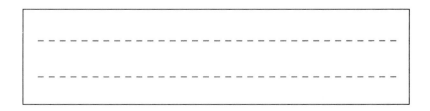

Fig. 9.12 Types of working relationships to encourage in my group are...

You could do this with other colleagues to get a consensus of opinion of one of your groups. Or as part of a training exercise, you could build up views of what to encourage in a new group.

Similarly, what type of relationships do you want to discourage? Select a group you are, or were, a part of and make a note of what you don't want. You could do this as a small group activity based on your collective experiences (see Fig. 9.13).

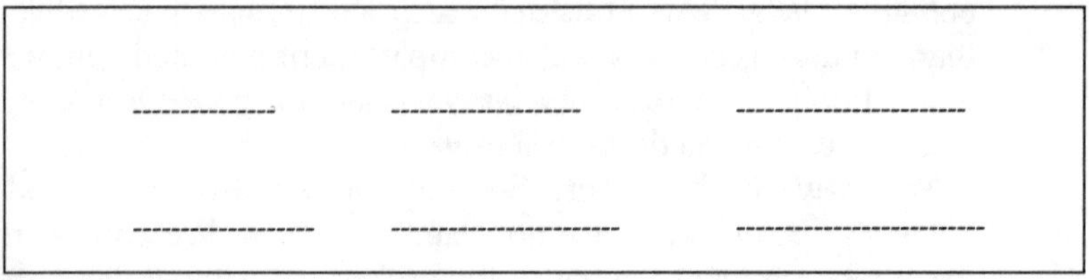

Fig. 9.13   Types of working relationships we don't want to encourage.

Some patterns of relationships that you want to discourage are:

- excessive competition (of the win–lose type),
- excessive self-protective behaviour,
- collusive ways of working,
- combative destructive patterns,
- self-idealizing,
- idealization of the profession or the organization.

The common element in the list above is that they seek to impose patterns of working that restrict the openness of interaction between people. Essentially these are defensive communicative strategies. They are intended to protect those who promote them from threats they see, or anticipate. Whether real or imagined, the impact of these worries are tangible so far as those who hold them are concerned.

If you see evidence of these types of behaviour beginning to predominate in your group you must find out what is going on to cause these reactions, check to see if it is just your perception and decide what to do in response.

In contrast, more productive work relationships often seem to flourish where a very different set of phenomena are present. Where, for example:

- there is a climate of allowing dissent and working with it,
- each person is seen as valuable and is encouraged to contribute,
- the quality of the working environment is recognized as important,
- colleagues work with and for each other,

- corporate cohesion and belief exists,
- learning from experience is valued
- lack of perfection is not penalized.

The relationship criteria that is predominant can significantly affect the working climate and culture of the group, team or meeting. The relationship dimension sets the tone for how groups will go about their work and the quality of that group as an entity.

5. Developing a culture of mutual respect and regard

How you treat me has a direct effect on how I feel about you and what I will or will not willingly do for you at work. How we treat each other can affect our psychological well-being and our work achievements. Not everyone takes this position, but if I feel badly treated or ignored by you I cannot but be affected by your behaviour towards me. Try as I might to put it out of my mind it will continue to lurk somewhere and have some influence on our future relationship.

This does not mean that I need to be treated with caution or that I am over-sensitive. It does mean that I believe I have a right to be acknowledged and treated with appropriate regard and value by others. In turn, I intend to do likewise in my dealings with others.

More publicity is now being given to the importance of building and sustaining effective and constructive work relationships. There is an increasing acknowledgement that technical expertise alone, in whatever field, is *not* enough to be successful at work.

Nowhere is this more important than in situations where the work is centred around people in need of care and who may be in trauma. The relationship between care advice and medical intervention, the cared-for and the carer assumes enormous significance. Health care settings are some of the most difficult to work in. The intense emotional nature of the nurse–patient relationship exerts a major influence on the perceptions of patients, relatives, and carers. Much of this comes from building and sustaining a culture of mutual respect and regard. Also it comes from a belief that we are there to do the best we can even though the circumstances are difficult, traumatic and trying.

On the home visit, in the clinic, and on the ward there is a clear focus on what needs to be done for the patient or the client. This invariably revolves around the professional collaboration of the carers and the maintenance of respect and regard between them (see Fig. 9.14).

Figure 9.14 shows the patient at the centre as the primary focus around which the others revolve. This is both in relation to each other and the patient. This collaboration around the patient, recognizing that each has a contribution to make, leads to a sustaining, mutually respectful working culture. When the central patient focus becomes lost, or moves out of focus, this can result in the dissolution of the cohesive pattern shown in Fig. 9.14.

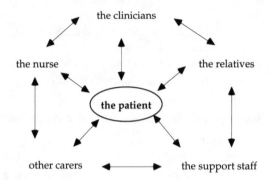

the clinicians

the nurse

the relatives

the patient

other carers

the support staff

Fig. 9.14   Working for the patient.

The same pattern of professional collaboration, insight and skills applied to clinical work, based on mutual trust and regard, is also needed when teams get together in the meeting room. Too rarely however, have I experienced the collaboration, collective wisdom, insight and problem solving shown in everyday clinical work carried forward into the administrative and business dimensions of the nurse's work.

It may be that the critical combination of sensitivity and skill in providing direct patient care is seen as not necessary in non-direct care situations. If this is the case, much is lost. It is likely that business and professional meetings will be less well managed than they should be. The *esprit de corps* that is generated in direct care situations is less likely to be generated in group and business meeting settings.

A recognition of the skills and competencies that each person brings and uses with others can create and sustain a culture of mutual respect and regard. If for some reason these abilities and sensitivities are not utilized it is difficult to develop the necessary productive and supportive work culture. Because of the overwhelming emphasis placed on task completion as the 'real' work to be done, less attention is normally given to relationship building in health care work.

The importance of how we treat each other at work cannot be overemphasized. It impacts on all aspects of our life. How we relate to our patients and our colleagues, and in turn how they relate to and treat us is enormously important. It determines what we will be able to achieve together and how we feel about ourselves and our abilities.

Usually, the emphasis for the nurse is firmly placed on the immediate clinical task to be done. But it will be as much about *how* the dressing is applied as it is being changed, that the patient will take strength and support from. It may be that the qualitative care the patient receives helps them through another day just as much as the completion of a specified clinical task.

Being competent, professional, energetic and a sound thinker is all very well, but much of your success and professionalism will be based on your attitude to others. Being respectful and having a positive regard of others, despite differences of opinion, will enable you to keep in place a sound foundation on which to develop for the future.

6. Achieving the intended results

The earlier five components all build up to this one: the results we want to achieve. This is where they all come together and where the other dimensions considered bear fruit. If the other parts are in place you should achieve the purposes outlined for your endeavours. If not, expect problems and difficulties along the way.

The results are at the centre of Fig. 9.15. All the other facets introduced are geared to achieving the work set out in the first place.

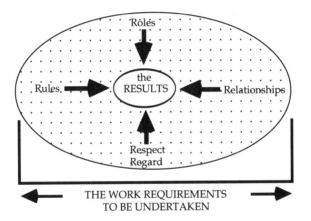

Fig. 9.15 The six 'R' framework for group working.

This framework (the six-'Rs') can be used as a way of remembering six very critical areas to think about when in groups, teams or meetings. When you have the opportunity to set up a new work group, or meeting, or are given the job of reviewing the performance of an existing team you could use these headings as the basis for your review. If, on the other hand, you already have a different way of looking at groups use these ideas to add your own or to build up your own framework combining all the ingredients that work for you.

References

Dixon, N. (1979) *On the Psychology of Military Incompetence*, Futura, London.

Harvey, J. (1988) *The Abilene Paradox*, Lexington Books, Lexington, MA.

Janis, I. (1982) *Groupthink*, Houghton Mifflin Co., Boston, MA.

Chapter 10
Groups and Their Dynamics

This chapter considers some of the dynamics that occur in groups and some of the ways in which groups themselves develop as entities. The last part of the chapter refocuses attention on to some of the formalized roles in groups as opposed to the generic ones covered in Chapter 9.

Even though you may have considered all the points suggested in Chapter 9 there is no guarantee that the group, team or the meeting will be a productive gathering. Try as you might to encourage mutual regard and internal cohesion, it may elude you. You may be unable to control all the dynamics that come into play when a group forms. For example, as soon as you join that group you will bring your background experiences with you, much of which will have been in groups or gatherings of one kind or another. Some collective dynamics will immediately start to function as a result of *this* unique group being together.

You will see similarities and differences between those present in the group and people you have worked with in the past. This will lead you to make assumptions about working with these people on the basis of little data. You will do this consciously or unconsciously with every member of the group. You will be prone to gravitate to some members and to avoid or distance yourself from others. From some you are likely to accept what they say whereas with others you may disagree. These reactions are the effects of your internal dynamics, drawing on earlier experiences you have had of similar people elsewhere. These are called *individual dynamic* processes.

When the group starts to function scenarios will be enacted that trigger memories of past events and words will be said in ways that may hold a deeply personal meaning. This may lead you to over-react, oppose, or in other ways work less productively with the group than you had originally intended. You will not necessarily have total influence over some of these feelings and reactions. They will unexpectedly surge through you and affect your behaviour and your perceptions of what is happening. These are called the *group dynamics* processes.

When thinking about group situations you need, if you don't do this already, to look at them in a multidimensional way to understand more fully what may be happening. This applies to clinical situations, professional meetings, social settings, etc. However I am not suggesting you look at every grouping in such detail as this chapter makes possible. For a start you will overload yourself; secondly you may become too intense; and thirdly it might reduce your ability to enter fully into the work you are there to do. The way to use these ideas about groups, teams and meetings is a little at a time – not try to apply them all in one go.

Enabling a group to work well and effectively is a complex business. It needs attention given to the following emphases and interactions:

- *Emphasis 1:* the *formal tasks* set for that group/meeting to complete,
- *Emphasis 2:* an integration of the *different personalities* involved,
- *Emphasis 3:* use of meetings *procedures and practices* to structure the group's work,
- *Emphasis 4:* sensitivity and understanding the *group's dynamic processes.*

The focus for this chapter is on *emphasis 4.* This concerns the group's dynamic processes which can be collectively as well as individually driven. The trouble is that so much of what goes on dynamically cannot be seen, touched or proven. Because it is emotionally charged, it is very rarely openly acknowledged or talked about. All we know is that the effect of the dynamics in groups is very real and very powerful. I hope the next few pages will give you some 'hand-holds' to get a grip of some of it!

Frames and levels of behaviour in groups

When you are in a group you should remember that you cannot see everything that is going on. You and your colleague participants will react differently – and from moment to moment – depending on whether or not your needs are being met and how you are being treated in that group.

There are a number of different levels of activity going on simultaneously in the group.

- behaviour driven by individual and collective motivations,
- individual behaviour related to the task or to their self,
- work on material that is not always available to all present.

It is a complicated and web-like situation. These three dimensions of behaviour and interaction within the group create a very complex arena within which to work and remain effective.

Ideally Fig. 10.1, which should really be in 3-D, shows these features together. The vertical axis extends from material that is there to be seen, discussed and explored in the group (the *manifest* work of the group) through to material which is only known to some and is withheld from others (the *covert* group's workings) and then includes material which we are not consciously aware of but which will influence what occurs (the *unconscious* group processes).

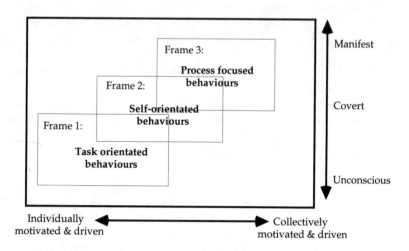

Fig. 10.1   A model of group processes and dynamics.

The horizontal axis shows the range between individually driven activities and those which are collectively owned and shared by the group. No doubt you can recall examples in a group where at times there is just one member of the group trying to push through their idea or perspective but where, in different ways, everyone else is resisting this. That person's idea may be relevant, realistic and helpful but the majority have decided on an alternative, possibly foolish, option. Conversely, you will know how very different it is when the whole group gets hold of an idea and goes with it. This can be quite worrying because the group, riding on the wave of its collective 'high', can get out of control and lose touch with reality and makes decisions when in such a condition, with disastrous results.

During this each member, in their thinking and their behaviour, is balancing the three different sets of behaviours shown in the middle of Fig. 10.1. They are in the middle because they will be influenced by the vertical and horizonal influences just described. In the middle we can be:

(1) working to help the formal work get done, or
(2) more concerned to secure our own personal position and standing, or
(3) working in ways that will facilitate effective group functioning.

Each of these will probably fluctuate between three orientations throughout the meeting and they will guide our thinking and influence our behaviour.

Figure 10.1 offers quite a number of ways of looking at how meetings function. We can never hope to have a full grasp of all the interactions and influences in play at any one time, yet we can get a good idea of what is being played out even if we cannot grasp all the details.

Two ideas strike me as significant here. The first is that you can get caught up in collective *group dynamics*, the type of situation where you find yourself going along with the flow when, at the same time, you are aware of hesitation, doubt or resistance in your actions. The second is that what you see in front of you is unlikely to be the full story. There will invariably be other influences at play of which you are unaware, either because you choose to not acknowledge them or because they are operating at an *unconscious level.*

If you think back to recent meetings you could use Fig. 10.1 to build up an idea of what may have been going on as the meeting progressed. Most important of all you can think back to how your involvement altered and what made you operate in different ways at different times in the same meeting.

Captured by the group?

As an experienced and professionally trained adult, how would you feel if I suggested that sometimes you are *captured by the group* you are working in? That try as you might you find yourself unable to use your skills and abilities freely in voicing your opinions. That you were somehow stopped from participating in what was going on around you. That on the contrary you get caught up in, and pulled along by, the flow of things which at one level seem to be purposeful and pro-ductive, but which leaves you with a nagging doubt that all is not as it should be.

I can recall times when I have experienced such feelings and felt a little dismayed, when I later reflected upon it. I have been disappointed in myself that I did not act differently. It was because it would have been such a struggle to have done so, and . . . well, it was easier to go with the flow at the time.

What may have been happening was that the group had begun working on an emotional basis that, unconsciously, influenced every-body present to conform to a pattern of working which at that time met some unstated needs of that group. This possibility sounded worrying the first time I came across it some years ago. However, having watched groups in action, I have reflected on my own behaviour in a group (team or meeting) and unexpected things do happen. I vividly recall my experiences, over several years, on one management team where at one level we seemed to be very hard working. We were dedicated to the task of running the health district, and yet very little was actually achieved. Much was explained later when I learnt about the ideas of Bion (1961) and his model of unconscious group processes.

Bion was a psychoanalyst who introduced revolutionary ideas about what happens in groups based on his experience with military therapy groups. He observed that when groups form for work, there are unconscious emotional disturbances and obstacles that make work on the formal tasks of the group difficult to progress.

He didn't know why this was but suggested that unconscious patterns of group cohesion form which then interfere with the tasks and purposes set out for them to accomplish. He linked the trigger that activates these defensive behaviours to a sense of anxiety or some threat picked up within the group and which then, for a period, dominates the group's dynamics.

Now the really interesting thing is that such unconscious patterns form and present themselves as seemingly acceptable and appropriate ways of working. On the surface the work group may appear to work effectively even though what may be driving the behaviours, which are actually counter-productive, remains obscure. He identified three distinct patterns: dependency, pairing and fight–flight. These lead a group to believe it is functioning productively, as if all is going well. It is 'as if' all those present were working from a common but unstated assumption about what they as a group should be doing.

Bion differentiates between a group that freely utilizes the talents of those present (a *sophisticated* work group) from one which gets diverted by these strong unconscious dynamics which he calls a *basic assumption* group. He suggests that every group is prone to episodes of 'basic assumption' workings and that the best one can do is to minimize such periods and maximize the group's 'sophisticated work' functioning.

From his observations and experiences he discerned three basic assumptions that regularly take over the behaviour of groups:

- the basic assumption of 'dependency',
- the basic assumption of 'pairing',
- the basic assumption of 'fight–flight'.

The basic assumption of dependency: is a group which meets around a leader on whom it depends for nourishment and protection. The dynamic here is a kind of corporate madness in which every member colludes and stifles independent thought or cooperative work. It is as if the only person worth listening to is the boss.

The basic assumption of pairing: is altogether different. It is centred on an almost mystical belief that collaboration between (any) two of the members of the team will create a solution to the preoccupations, problems and concerns of the group. The rest of the group finds they are unable to contribute, and let the pair sort it all out.

The fight–flight assumption: maintains the view and perspective that the work of the group is one of the following. Either to confront and fight something (i.e. the problems and pressures impacting on the group) or to seek to escape from the matters of concern and threat as quickly as possible. In this mode the 'leader' becomes the person who offers the ways and means of acting on these defensive impulses and directing the group's fight or flight behaviour.

When a group is working from these basic assumptions little constructive work is actually being achieved although at the time it may seem as if a great deal of productive work is going on. It may seem as if real collaboration and progress is being made, yet afterwards you find yourself wondering exactly what was achieved. Therein lies the lure and the seduction of these patterns of group working. It can feel very positive, energetic and busy, but it is a 'busyness' aimed at denying the actual issues and work to be done. It is energy channelled to defend or deny work the group should face up to and confront.

At first sight this may all appear to be a little far-fetched and fanciful. You can test these notions against your own experiences. Focus on one or two of the groups you are a part of, either in or out of health care, where you meet on a regular basis. Now . . .

- Can you recall meetings where you felt unable to get involved, or you felt as if you were an onlooker? All you could do was listen to an intense discussion between two of your colleagues and where the remainder of the group seemed to allow these two to create the solution (pairing?).
- What about situations where the only criteria was how to stop the administration reducing the staffing levels (fight–flight?).
- There may have been episodes where you all expected the leader of the group to provide the resolution; that if we only show enough deference and support she will see us through (dependency?).

The reason why these basic assumption patterns are dysfunctional is that they delude the group into believing the group is fully functioning and using its collective capabilities reasonably well. However this is the opposite of what is occurring. In these three different ways the capabilities of the group are not being called upon in an equal way. Most will feel that they are somehow unable to contribute as fully as they could. They will feel that there are invisible blocks and barriers operating, and that the group is becoming too inward oriented for its own good. Yet the problem is that individually they may find themselves unable to intervene because the unstated and unconscious group pressure to go along with these patterns when they occur.

These patterns are not unusual or irrational. Bion sees them as an inevitable part of group life and in that sense they are normal and to be expected to occur and recur. The mark of an effective group is how it copes with and handles these aspects of its workings, and its success in achieving a productive balance between *basic assumption* group and *sophisticated* work group behaviour when it is then engaging more fully the talents of all the group for the tasks that group is there to perform.

You need to be aware that such processes exist and that they, temporarily at least, can take over you and your group. They can divert the efforts of the group away from its tasks and towards these defensive preoccupations.

Groupthink

Sometimes it becomes extremely difficult to behave freely as you can see from the *basic assumption* material which is being driven subconsciously. Sometimes it is very difficult to think differently to those around you, even when everyone has been fully involved and had their say. This can happen to such an extent that to even consider raising doubts, or offer an alternative strategy feels like a betrayal of trust of one's colleagues. Where it could be seen as evidence of a personal misjudgement of the highest order.

Over a period of time with a close knit group of colleagues it is easy to be trapped into thinking that 'we know best, we are the best and the rest of the world is downright wrong!' Pride in a group's work or worthwhile changes are to be commended, of course but situations can arise where it becomes almost impossible to question the value or appropriateness of what your group is contemplating doing. That is when things get dangerous and can go badly wrong.

Examples of how this happens, at the highest levels, are given by Irving Janis (1982) who coined the word 'Groupthink' to describe this type of inward looking group thinking. He used as an example the ill-judged decision of President Kennedy to invade Cuba in 1962 (the Bay of Pigs invasion). He suggested

> The more amiability and *esprit de corps* among the members of a policy-making in-group, the greater is the danger that independent critical thinking will be replaced by groupthink, which is likely to result in irrational and dehumanising actions directed against out-groups.

He does not suggest that all groups with a strong sense of collaboration and mutual support suffer from 'groupthink', but that caution is needed to minimize its tendency. Pressure from colleagues who share your views, values and overall objectives to conform to the plan being presented are difficult to resist. But this can lead to an inward looking conformity that (temporarily at least) loses touch with the wider practical realities. It can result in decisions being made that have catastrophic consequences.

Janis examined cases of historic fiascos and identified eight main symptoms that run through them.

Type 1: Over-estimations of the group – its power and morality

(1) An illusion of invulnerability, shared by most or all the members, which creates excessive optimism and encourages the taking of extreme risks.
(2) An unquestioned belief in the group's inherent morality (we are right, the others must be wrong), inclining the members to ignore the ethical or moral consequences of their decisions.

Type II: Closed-mindedness

(3) Collective efforts to rationalize in order to discount warnings or other information that might lead members to reconsider their assumptions before they recommit themselves to their past policy decisions.
(4) Stereotyped views of enemy leaders as too evil to warrant genuine attempts to negotiate, or as too weak or stupid to counter whatever risky attempts are made to defeat their purposes.

Type III: Pressures toward uniformity

(5) Self-censorship of deviations from the apparent group consensus, reflecting each member's inclination to minimize the importance of his doubts and counter-arguments.
(6) A shared illusion of unanimity concerning judgements conforming to the majority view (partly resulting from self-censorship of deviations, augmented by the false assumption that silence means consent).
(7) Direct pressure on any member who expresses strong arguments against any of the group's stereotypes, illusions, or commitments, making clear that this type of dissent is contrary to what is expected of all loyal members.
(8) The emergence of self-appointed 'mind-guards' – members who protect the group from adverse information that might shatter their shared complacency about the effectiveness and morality of their decisions (see Janis 1982, pp. 174–5).

How often have you noticed or even taken a lead in prompting the actions Janis has identified. Think back over your experiences and use Fig. 10.2 to chart what you recall. You will need to guard against these adverse behaviours in the groups in which you are working.

If Janis' work seems accurate, you should be able to work through these 'symptoms' and see to what extent they were part of your experiences.

These processes of a group almost taking over its members are very

	rarely - occasionally - often - always
Type I: Over estimations of the group	
illusion of invulnerability	
unquestioned moral beliefs	
Type II: Closed mindedness	
collective rationalisation	
negative stereotyping	
Type III: Pressures towards uniformity	
self censorship of own differences	
shared illusion of unanimity	
pressure on dissenters to conform	
filtering out of contrary external information	

Fig. 10.2   Watching out for 'groupthink' symptoms.

real as are instances where ambiguity about what the group really wants to do can lead to fruitless and expensive misuse of resources. In his book *The Abilene Paradox* (which is subtitled 'compassionate insights into the craziness of organisational life') Jerry Harvey (1988) considers, through a series of brief *user-friendly* essays, that 'the theory and practice of organisation and management frequently reflects convoluted thought processes and that each member runs the risk of living their organisational lives in quiet desperation, trapped in decaying organisations'. Strong stuff: yet the experiences he recounts may be familiar to you at work.

He draws attention to how everyday experiences at work can gather momentum and take on lives of their own. This can be despite the fact that few, if any, people want to take part in them. His research covers a wide range of organizations. He has called this dysfunction the 'Abilene Paradox' where 'individuals frequently feel as if they are experiencing coercive organisational pressures to conform when they actually are responding to the dynamics of mismanaged agreement'.

In his book Harvey recounts how a family group embarked on a journey – to Abilene on a hot dusty Sunday – which no one really wanted to go on but where each thought their companions did. At the end of a long, boring, pointless trip in uncomfortable conditions, it emerged they would each have preferred to stay home. However, no one had been prepared to say what they wanted or been willing to handle the reactions of the others. They assumed these reactions would be hostile. In the end, all was wasted and no one was satisfied. Can you think of any parallels from your experiences?

These situations arise through not expressing your genuine view about an issue to be resolved or a suggestion that has been made. Harvey suggests that much of the behaviour in organisations, previously thought of as reflecting conformity pressures, could really be an expression of a collective anxiety. Behaviour like this serves as a defence against taking a lead or making a stand. When people do this it can lead to unproductive collective behaviour, wasted time and effort, a foolish use of resources and lower morale. He suggests that rather than face up to issues we prefer to go along with less risky options, which can lead us to less fulfilling outcomes.

Models of group development

Some group behaviour relates to the stage of development of the group itself. If it has only recently been formed it will be preoccupied by different concerns to those of a group that has been working together for some months, or years even. Just as we change as we get older so do groups. This can explain why sometimes a group cannot initially seem able to take on board ideas or ways of working yet several meetings later it finds them acceptable. I am not suggesting that a newly formed group cannot produce quality work, but that it takes time and maturity to increase its capabilities.

Over a period of time it is likely that a group will be more confident. They will produce results that are qualitatively more than the sum of the abilities of each of the members put together. This 'coming together' takes time. There appear to be stages of development that groups (teams, meetings) need to go through before they can become fully productive and operational.

Tuckman's four stage model

One of the best known models of group development was developed from Bruck Tuckman's (1965) research into the stages of small group development. He proposed four general stages of development through which groups progress. Rather like Erikson's model (see Chapter 5) each carries particular difficulties that need to be confronted and substantially resolved before the group can move on to the next stage of operational development. This is not to suggest that a group won't do any work unless they have resolved all the issues, but that the effectiveness and the quality of their work will not be as good as it should be until they have tackled those issues.

Tuckman suggests that there are four stages of group functioning: *forming, storming, norming* and *performing.* They chart a progression

Stage 1 – the Forming Stage: When new groups form – and this applies to an informal coming together of four or five people – there is invariably some anxiety and some confusion about how this group of people will be able to work together. This is especially so if new people join others who have previously worked together and who will have generated their own ways of working and can be expected to want these to continue even though there are new members.

There is anxiety, confusion and uncertainty as members try to decide how they will work together and what structure to use to organise themselves. A major issue is 'where do I fit in?', 'who are the others?', and 'what is going to happen here?' Initial politeness and superficial acquiescent behaviours will begin to change as people start to test out what is acceptable or not and find their feet. Bids for roles etc. will begin to be made but politely.

Stage 2 – the Storming Stage: This stage is reached when the group has clarified what is to be done and where members have begun to establish how the work is to be undertaken. It is from that position that increasingly open attacks and challenges are made by members about who does what and why, of challenges to the leadership and dissension and conflict within the team.

There is tension, confrontation and disharmony. Testing the norms established so far and 'getting involved' characterise this phase of the group's existence – much seems under threat and challenge. Members are no longer polite. How the tensions, conflicts of interest, disagreements are handled and then resolved has a major influence on the work culture of the group and determines how they behave to each other subsequently.

Stage 3 – the Norming Stage: This stage presupposes that agreements have been reached about many task and process matters that will determine what we do and how we work together. The climate will be co-operative rather than competing or conflictual, although difficulties will still arise. We will have agreed norms of behaviour relevant to the work we have to do and are likely to be more sensitive to the needs of the individual members of the group.

There may still be difficulties to be resolved but some progress in agreeing
ways of working more effectively together will have been made. Problems can
crop up if there are unresolved matters hanging over from the Storming stage
which may stop some members from releasing their full potential. Therefore as
the group develops its ways of being with, and of working with, each other it is
prudent to allow unresolved issues, concerns and feelings from earlier stages
to be expressed and then addressed.

Stage 4 – the Performing Stage: To have reached this stage will have taken some
time and it will describe a group that is both task focused and sensitive to the
individual wants and needs of its members. The culture of the group will be
open and able to sustain – and use constructively – disagreements and
problems when they occur to make the group more effective.

The members will be fully involved and committed, able to sort out problems
as they arise and realistic about its performance and accomplishments.

Fig. 10.3   Outline of Tuckman's model of group development.

from a group of individuals thrust together to a productive and integrated
team. The main facets of the four stages are shown in Fig. 10.3.

Movement through the stages takes time. It will be different for each
group of people and regression to an earlier stage of group development can be precipitated by a group crisis (such as the loss of a key
member or a change to the primary tasks of the group). This then
necessitates the group re-establishing aspects of their work together that
had previously been resolved. Figure 10.4 shows aspects of this group
development.

The model does not suggest that you have to wait until stages three or
four before a group begins to be productive. However, for any group to
become optimally effective it needs to have addressed and resolved the
types of issues indicated in Fig. 10.3. The model suggests that unless
these concerns are aired and worked out they will preoccupy and impair
group working.

Given this brief introduction where would you say the groups of
people you work with are in terms of Tuckman's model? Use the
material in Fig. 10.3 as a guide to the types of preoccupations experienced by group members. This will give you a clue as to where the group
may be in this development sequence (see Fig. 10.5).

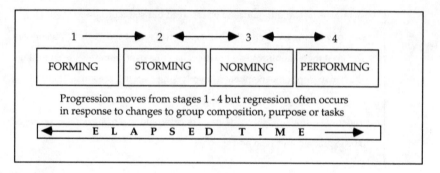

Fig. 10.4 Tuckman's stages of group development.

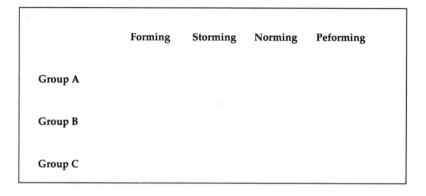

Fig. 10.5 Relating Tuckman's model to your experience.

You may like to continue to assess how your groups progress over the next few months. Keep an eye out to see what happens in the group when the *status quo* gets disturbed in some way, for example changes to members, changes to the brief of the group, performance criteria adjustments, additional (or fewer) tasks, etc.

It is helpful to remember that *all* groups go through similar stages of development to those noted by Tuckman. The very least you can do therefore, is be prepared for the differing emphases which Tuckman suggests will arise. For example, don't be obsessed by the storming characteristics, or too lulled into the initial forming stage characteristics.

Underlying all these development processes will be the work that each group or team must complete. This should be the spur to the development and maintenance – not group cohesion alone. The work to be done should dictate the size, shape, priorities and continuity of the group.

Gibb's model – characteristics of group climate

In contrast Gibb's model of group development focuses on the concerns of the individual members (see Gibb, 1971). These critically affect the performance of that person, and through them, the whole team. He suggests that in all group interactions there are four 'primary social needs' that determine an individual's behaviour. When these are not met sufficiently other, less functional, behaviours are likely to emerge and impede effective group performance.

Figure 10.6 sets out the core ideas of his approach. What is helpful is the way the basic needs of the members of the team are set out. They are concerns and considerations that reflect the types of worries most people take with them into a group setting. If this is so, why isn't more attention given to these concerns at an early stage in the proceedings to try to reduce some of the anxieties that are linked to the four core needs for:

● acceptance
● communication
● clear objectives
● control.

If this were done more often it may result in colleagues working more freely, productively and confidently together. The model is shown in Fig. 10.6.

Primary Needs of group members	Underlying consideration	Behaviour if need met	Behaviour if need not met
Acceptance	membership	acceptance confidence trust	suspicion mistrust fear
Communication	decisions	spontaneity openness	caution polite facade
Clear Objectives	productivity	creative work cooperation commitment	apathy competition
Control	organisation	joint problem-solving. flexible roles, inter-dependent working	dependency & counter-dependency rivalry

Fig. 10.6 Outline of Gibb's model of group development.

These dimensions highlight what you may be looking for to make you feel part of a group. The table suggests what the behavioural consequences for the group may be if your needs for acceptance, communication, clear objectives, and control were met or not.

Often we concentrate on the positive and the disruptive behaviour we see in our colleagues without usually, thinking about why they may be behaving in this way. The Gibb model suggests some of the underlying needs that we bring with us into a group and it is how well or not we feel these are met that then causes us to behave as we do. For example, just because I behave in a non-constructive way in the group does not necessarily mean that I am being awkward for the sake of it. My behaviour may indicate that my needs are not being met, or being denied, and this is how I am alerting you to this.

The most productive way of responding therefore, is not to penalize me, or coerce me to behave as you want me to, but to find out *why* I am disagreeing, or behaving in a difficult manner. Think back to the push–pull influencing model. You may identify a need that still needs to be met. If this can be identified we can then work on it together.

Select two or three groups that you are a part of and note the concerns and issues that affect you as a member. Relate these to the Gibb model and see what is missing for you from that group. For example, is it acceptance, communication, clear objectives and/or control that is missing? Use Fig. 10.7 for your analysis.

	Acceptance	Communication	Objectives	Control
Group 1				
Group 2				
Group 3				

Fig. 10.7   Application of the Gibb model to my group membership.

This may help you to be clearer about your position in that group and if anything is missing. You may then be able to achieve or come to terms with what you are still looking for in that group. Also you will be able to see what options are available to improve your situation.

You can also use the model to see how those around you are relating to the group. For example, you could recall how colleagues behave in the group and look to see if there is any consistent pattern and if it fits into the Gibb framework. You may notice that colleagues consistently become concerned about similar matters, such as communication concerns. These may suggest that, to some extent, one or more of the primary concerns are not yet met sufficiently for them to work to the full in that group. It could be that they are stuck at one stage in the development of their relationship in that group, yet be unclear about what it is that concerns them and could be blocking their performance.

You may want to outline the model to them. See if it can help them identify any concerns they may have about the group. For example, acceptance or communication needs that remain unmet. This may help them resolve their concerns and allow them to participate more fully in that group.

Having done this you can consider doing the same for yourself. You too may be 'stuck' in some way in the group which is leading you to hold off, reduce your commitment, etc. You may be able to use 'Gibb' to deduce:

- your current group involvement issues,
- what needs to be changed for you to become more involved and engaged,
- if you want things to be different or to keep things as they are.

Whatever you decide, you now have another means of reflecting on what is happening and on your position. This gives you an opportunity to make a more informed choice about what to do now or in the future.

Roles in groups, teams and meetings

Creating a fully functioning team remains an elusive goal. The search for a way to achieve this has spawned a huge industry with questionnaires, books, tapes, training courses etc. Many of these offer ways to achieve 'the effective team'. Yet, how do you create the perfect team? One outcome has been an increasing interest in team roles. 'If we can get these sorted out then surely we'll have a peak performing team – won't we?'

There are two different approaches to looking at roles in groups and teams. One is to identify generic roles and behaviours to be covered if a team is to work well. The other is to identify and define specific roles needed in a team, and then to build up a team with these specific attributes in mind.

Much attention has been given to defining the core roles needed and then finding the appropriate mix. It is rather like mixing the ingredients for a cake. Roles become the institutionalized, and formally sanctioned channels for powerful dynamics within a group. They signify legitimized power and status. At one level the role of Chairperson, for example, is clearly set out and well-known – it will be described what tasks are involved for such a role. What is not known is *how*, in terms of the dynamics, that role will be exercised. This dimension of roles is not usually discussed but having a role is far more than just performing a specific set of responsibilities under a title. A formalized group role gives the opportunity to exert influence and affects the tensions and emotionality of the group. Neither the generic roles nor the specific roles fully explore these dimensions in groups.

Generic team roles

The focus here is on the types of roles and behaviours that are needed in any team, group and meeting to assist the completion of the work. I am assuming that the appropriate people should be present in the group and have the technical knowledge and experience needed for the work to be completed successfully.

With the right people involved each group then needs to pay attention to three different, but complementary, aspects of its functioning if that group is to achieve the best results. These are shown in Fig. 10.8.

---

1 **the Task Focus** : an emphasis on getting the work completed

2 **the Process Focus** : an emphasis on helping the group

actually work together (the emotions & dynamics)

3 **the Procedural Focus** adopting and managing suitable

methods and procedures for the group's work

Fig. 10.8   Three dimensions of group functioning.

Some examples of these three levels of group working are given in Fig. 10.9. While there is some overlap between the generic task and process roles, they do cover different aspects of a group's functioning.

From your experience in groups and in meetings where do you see the emphasis placed between these three facets of a group's functioning? As before, if you had 100 points how would you distribute them between the three to:

- reflect where the emphasis is placed,
- where you see most problems and difficulties occurring in groups and in meetings (see Fig. 10.10).

Most groups put their emphasis onto task achievement considerations and tend to pay a bit of attention to the procedures the group should follow. I rarely find that much attention is explicitly given to the process side of a group's functioning (the more dynamic and emotional side of things). Yet from my experience it is usually by not attending to the dynamics of a group that outstanding group performance is most impeded.

Task Focus	Process Focus	Procedural Focus
is about	is about	is about
setting targets	encouraging	what procedures to
summarising	diagnosing	follow in our work
recording	bringing others in	
giving information	summarising	what decision making
integrating ideas	finding common ground	and problem solving
evaluating	setting constructive tone	to adopt
making decisions	relationship building	sequence of work
diagnosing	energising	management of group
seeking information	building collaboration	

Fig. 10.9   Task, process and procedure examples.

1. Where I see the emphasis is placed in my experience of groups		2. Where do I see most problems in groups coming from	
on the Task	points	from Task issues	points
on the Process	points	from Process issues	points
on the Procedures	points	from Procedural issues	points
	100 points		100 points

Fig. 10.10   Where is the emphasis? Where do the problems occur?

You may like to monitor some future meetings and assess where the attention is being placed, and then note where the problems occur. You may realize that too little attention is being given to recording the decisions being reached or that the group also needs to decide how to manage its limited time etc. You could then look for ways of covering these procedural aspects more fully. Or it may be that problems in the group may not stem from the quality of the decisions being reached but in how this is being done. Paying more attention to the group process will then be the key to enhancing group performance.

Some examples of concerns that can emerge if too little attention is given to help the group function better together (the process side) are found in the following:

- unhelpful individual competition,
- resentment at the role a colleague may be taking which they wanted,
- being argumentative instead of asking for support,
- those who shout loudest get the attention,
- the quiet thinkers get overwhelmed and forgotten,
- subgroups emerge and the larger group can break up.

By being prepared to attend to concerns such as these we can help task accomplishment. By denying or neglecting them the whole group can be put at risk. Unless group process issues are addressed the work of the group can flounder completely, or at best, the final product is likely to be mediocre.

Most of our training and the terms of reference for our groups continue to emphasize task achievement. It is rare that they highlight the importance of building a collaborative group culture as a critical prerequisite for getting the work done. Yet often this is why groups fail to achieve their hoped-for goals.

I don't know how you assessed the relative weighting to the three dimensions in Fig. 10.10 but you probably put most of your points against task, a few against procedures and fewer still against process. In terms of where you thought the problems in groups occurred, you probably scored process a little higher and task as the highest. Figure 10.11 shows my estimate for comparison and discussion if necessary with colleagues.

I see the process (interactive and emotional) aspects of group working to be largely neglected yet it being that aspect of group working that, unless attended to, can totally disrupt and frustrate the work of a group.

Whereas it is normally expected that someone will take on a role in

1. Where I see the emphasis is placed in my experience of groups		2. Where do I see most problems in groups coming from	
on the Task	80 points	from Task issues	25 points
on the Process	5 points	from Process issues	55 points
on the Procedures	15 points	from Procedural issues	20 points
	100 points		100 points

Fig. 10.11   MJW's view.

directing the group in its task work (either as a chairperson, or task facilitator), or to handle the procedural side of things (time management, charting the discussion, providing a project plan, etc.) it is very unusual for anyone to take on, formally, the role of handling the process side of the group's work. Either this is because it is not thought necessary or it is expected that members themselves will informally, and intuitively, help the group work together. My experience is that this does not get done. Instead, skating over the issues, when sticking points arise, is far more frequent than addressing the underlying problems blocking the group's productivity.

One advantage of not specifying 'process' responsibilities is the flexibility and freedom it can give everyone to play a free role in helping the group function. A disadvantage is that there is no guarantee that these important dimensions of group working will be attended to in a rigorous way. This could leave the group vulnerable. The essential message from this section is that all three dimensions need to be attended to if the group is to be successful. If anyone is neglected the productivity of that group will suffer.

Specified team roles

The search for what makes a team successful has intrigued people for years. For some it is about how the team works and getting the balance right between, for example, task, process and procedures. For others it is about the composition of a team, designed so that each member brings very specific attributes which, when added together, will give an outstanding team.

Belbin's work (Belbin, 1981; 1993) is well known and often quoted in conversations about team roles. It is based on a careful examination of the behaviour of teams on Henley's senior management courses at Henley Management College. Belbin's model is based on observations and studies of teams and groups in action. He suggests that in addition to technical and functional expertise there are specific skills/orientations needed to produce well-founded, realistic and practical results to make the optimum use of the group's resources. He suggests that effective teams contain members with different blends of attributes, each of which is needed in the team, to varying extents, for it to be effective and work well. Belbin suggests that teams should be very carefully chosen with a balanced combination of different skills and approaches that, from his observations, make teams successful.

He identified eight specific roles briefly summarized in Fig. 10.12.

The intention is to create a balanced team and to avoid unhelpful duplication of roles. For example this can be where too many people vie for the role of chairman, or shaper, or where too few people are concerned with the role of completer–finisher. In reviewing the performance of an existing team the model can be used to identify the role

Outward Looking Roles	Inward Looking Roles
Chairman (CH) a critical role for the success of the team overall, calm leadership, will be self-confident and with average intellect,impartial, willing and able to listen, positive, relatively extravert [now called *Co-ordinator*]	**Company Worker (CW)** practical, tough-minded, disciplined approach to the work to be completed, conscientious [now called *Implementer*]
Plant (PL) the 'ideas people', individualistic, serious intent, impractical, intellectual, unorthodox, can be loners - can cause problems if too many in the team creative genius	**Monitor-Evaluator (ME)** evaluates proposals and pulls things together, detached, clear thinking, sober in approach, clever and shrewd, more impartial in assessing the team's work
Resource Investigator (RI) creative, pulls in ideas from outside the team, sociable, extravert, social skills, curious,	**Team Worker (TW)** works to keep the team functioning and reduce internal friction, sensitive to the internal dynamics, responsive rather decisive
Shaper (SH) similar role to Chairperson, high achievement motivation, impatient, challenging, provocative and can be disruptive, argumentative, a driving action-based leader	**Completer/Finisher (CF)** exercise the role of converting the team's 'good ideas' into practical outcomes, attention to detail, perseveres to an outcome, anxious, calm and consistent

Fig. 10.12 Outward and inward looking roles.

preference of members. It can also help identify where there are role gaps so that missing skills can then be brought into the team.

This is one way of looking at the disposition of roles needed in teams and of being more precise in what we want from the team. It can be unhelpful though, if the designations are used to label people and to box them into the role. The role titles are not neutral and it is, for example, probably more appealing to be labelled chairman or shaper than perhaps company worker or plant. This can lead to resentment and jealousy.

The most significant criticism of Belbin's work is that it was developed from watching teams chosen to do various tasks while on one of the Henley Management College's senior courses. So the field work was not based on real work teams and questions still remain of how viable his ideas are in practice. For the time being though, it remains one of the most prominent frameworks used to consider the composition of groups.

Individual commitment to the group

For many years I assumed that every member in a team or group shared a similar enthusiasm and commitment for the work undertaken. Now I realize this is a rather idealistic belief. Not everyone is committed to any one team, and a member's interest and attentiveness fluctuates during a meeting. I know this from my own experience and once I came to terms with this I began to look at how teams and groups worked with a new perspective. You might like to do the same.

First, decide which group, department or team to focus on. Think about the purpose and stated terms of reference and what actually goes on in that group and then consider:

- the extent to which each member is committed to the work of the group (you can do this by watching their behaviour),
- the degree of collaboration and subgrouping that you can observe within the group,
- from your observations, see if there are colleagues who do not seem to want to be in that group or to do the work.

Second, put these reflections into the format of Fig. 10.13 using the shape to represent the internal work environment of the group. 'W' is the main thrust and the formal remit of that group. Place the members (including yourself) on the diagram in relation to the group boundary. Show those who are very committed and in tune with the group's remit towards the centre of the shape and those less engaged towards the boundary.

You may feel that some of the group are half in and half out of the shape because they don't seem to want to be there or consider that they don't have a viable role to fulfil. There may be some members who are barely in the group at all – if so position them accordingly.

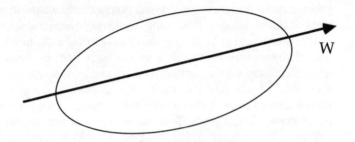

W   represents the Work of this particular group

Fig. 10.13   Plotting members' commitment to the group.

Having depicted your group members in the figure, see Fig. 10.14 as an example for you to review. 'A' is its leader. Before reading any further, have a look and make a few notes about this team. What messages come over to you? How integrated is this group? What are the key issues for the leader to address?

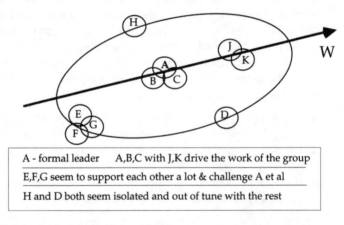

A - formal leader   A,B,C with J,K drive the work of the group
E,F,G seem to support each other a lot & challenge A et al
H and D both seem isolated and out of tune with the rest

Fig. 10.14   A hypothetical example.

It is clear that not everyone is uniformly committed to the work of the group ('W'). Some don't want to be there and are not interested in what is going on. Three of the group may be banding together in opposition to the formal leadership. There are two members who feel rather isolated and are probably ambivalent about being there at all. You probably have other observations as well.

This is a process you can use with your own groups. You can draw this type of diagram for each group you work in. Plot the members on it and see what observations you can make from each diagram. Some surprises may emerge. Your next step is to test out your thoughts to see if there is any evidence to support your assessments. Watch carefully what goes on in subsequent meetings.

This way of looking at things was a revelation to me. I stopped feeling so confused when things in group and team situations didn't go according to plan. I didn't feel annoyed with other members when they didn't seem to be as committed as I was to the work. I was able to look at things with a new perspective. I also felt less guilty when I sometimes lost interest in an item on the agenda.

This model makes it possible to assess the mood and behaviour of other members of a group in relation to the items under discussion and also to each other. It is hard to sustain a high level of interest if a meeting continues for very long. It is also unusual for everyone to be equally interested in every topic under discussion. Consequently, at any one time there will be some of the group paying less attention, and some may be taking a rest and speculating on their off-duty plans. They may be preoccupied with a patient under their care or 'resting' with their eyes open. Also some items are only of interest to a few of those present. Others will be thus less determined to influence the outcomes of the debate on these items.

By looking at a group in this way you are helped to predict where allegiances are formed and antipathies exist. You can get a sense of each person's 'distance' to or 'closeness' with each other. You can also get some sense of the individual, subgroup and whole group tensions and dynamics.

By observing groups carefully and with an informed eye you will be able to tell a great deal about what is happening. It can also help you to work more effectively and efficiently because you can then adopt a more perceptive and informed approach to your colleagues in the meeting. This can even be to the point of drawing them into the meeting if the need arises. You can also use this model as a planning device by speculating on a person's position on an issue and then assessing if you need others as backing prior to the next meeting. I have found it to be a straightforward and surprisingly helpful device.

References

Belbin, M. (1981) *Management Teams*, Heinemann, London.

Belbin, M. (1993) *Team Roles at Work*, Butterworth Heinemann, Oxford.

Bion, W.R. (1961) *Bion and Group Psychotherapy*, Experiences in Groups, Tavistock Publications, London.

Gibb, J.R. (1971) The effects of human relations training in: *Handbook of Psychotherapy and Behaviour Change* (Eds. A. Bergin and S. Garfield), Wiley, New York.

Harvey, J. (1987) *The Abilene Paradox*, Lexington Books, Lexington, MA.

Janis, I. (1982) *Groupthink*, 2nd edn, Houghton Mifflin Co., Boston, MA.
Tuckman, B. (1965) Developmental sequence in small groups. *Psychological Bulletin*, **63**, 6.

Further reading

Dixon, N. (1979) *On the Psychology of Military Incompetence*, Macdonald, London.
Douglas, T. (1976) *Groupwork Practice*, Tavistock Publications, London.
Dyer, W. (1977) *Team Building*, Addison-Wesley, Reading, MA.
Hinshelwood, R. (1987) *What happens in Groups*, Free Association Press, London.
Huczynski, A. and Buchanan, D. (1985) *Organizational Behaviour*, Prentice-Hall, London.
Morgan, G. (1986) *Images of Organization*, Sage Publications, London.
Pines, M. (1985) Routledge and Kegan Paul, London.
Rackham, N. and Morgan, T. (1977) *Behaviour Analysis in Training*, McGraw-Hill, Maidenhead.
Smith, P. (1973) *Groups within Organizations*, Harper & Row, London.
Sampson, E. and Marthas, M. (1977) *Group Process for the Health Professions*, Wiley, New York.
Williams, A. (1991) *Forbidden Agendas*, Routledge and Kegan Paul, London.
Weisbord, M. (1989) *Productive Workplaces*, Jossey-Bass Publishers, San Francisco.

Chapter 11
Leadership and Management

As a professional carer, irrespective of your formal job role, you are in a leadership role in a health care setting whether you want to be or not. People will look to you for guidance, advice, enthusiasm, belief, confirmation and support. They will also want to know about how, when, what, if, why and where things will happen. Again they will expect you to know about the monitoring of their progress, what the figures (and the words) mean and how well they are doing.

Much is expected of you. The least you can do is to accept the challenge and find out a little more about responding to the non-clinical aspects of the needs just noted above.

This chapter is about two prominent aspects of organizational life: *leadership* and *management*. Aspects of these are very similar to the needs expected of you in the last paragraph. The terms are often talked about as if they are the same and are regularly used interchangeably even though they refer to very different sets of behaviours. These differences are described in this chapter along with several theories about leadership and management that you will be able to use in your work.

In health care settings some of your most important followers will be your patients, their relatives, other non-clinically trained staff, colleagues more junior to yourself and colleagues more senior to you but who are less experienced than you in your specialty. Do not mistake the lack of a formal leadership title as not having leadership responsibilities – you do and not only for yourself but for others too.

Working in a formalized organization – such as in health care – with many different professions and grades of staff can lead you to equate leadership with a role on a hierarchy or a particular job title. However, from your own experience you will know that it is not like that at all. Each of us is a leader and through our example we influence the behaviour of others. We may not always influence them in the direction we had hoped for, but nevertheless the influence is still there.

Finally, you are a leader for yourself and no one else can do that for you, even though you will be influenced by people and situations around you.

The meaning of leadership and management

A prominent writer in this field suggests that *management* is about coping with the complexity of large organizations (Kotter, 1982) and that without management practices and procedures organizations would tend to become chaotic in ways that would threaten their very existence. By contrast, Kotter sees *leadership* as coping with change, an ability brought to prominence as a result of the ever increasing rates of change, competition and turbulence of modern industrial life. He defines management as organizing and ordering complexity (a more inward directed, micro focus). Leadership is about handling changing situations (a more outward looking, macro focus).

Both focuses are needed and there are overlaps between them. However *management* is more about order and effective control. *Leadership* is more about setting overall direction in response to changing circumstances as summarized in Fig. 11.1.

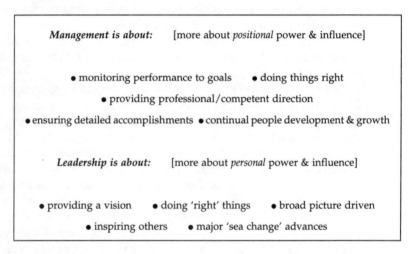

Management is about: [more about *positional* power & influence]

- monitoring performance to goals   • doing things right
- providing professional/competent direction
- ensuring detailed accomplishments • continual people development & growth

Leadership is about: [more about *personal* power & influence]

- providing a vision   • doing 'right' things   • broad picture driven
- inspiring others   • major 'sea change' advances

Fig.; 11.1 Leadership and management.

A central difference between leadership and management is defining the base of influence. For management it is more of a *positional* influence that drives the role. This includes:

- setting plans,
- monitoring progress,
- keeping things going,
- responding to the difficulties and problems that arise,
- giving good constructive support on very specific matters etc.

All of this can be done in a very inspirational and developmental, or procedural and administrative manner.

The influencing base for effective leadership is different. It is centred in the person and here it is the more *personal* characteristics that make the difference. These can engage, inspire, confirm and enable others to do outstanding work as shown in Fig. 11.2.

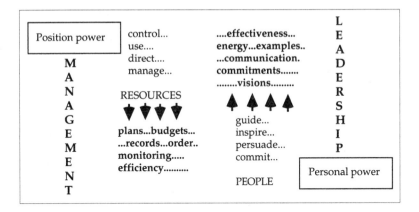

Fig. 11.2 The bases of leadership and management influence.

Which do you believe is the more important given these two linked, but fundamentally different, aspects of organization? Perhaps you feel that the differences noted above are rather artificial and there is no difference at all, that it is all 'management', or all 'leadership'.

Your views on this are important because they will affect:

- what you expect from others when they talk about *leadership* in the health care team, or management of the clinic,
- the performance criteria you use to assess others (for example, I could be a poor leader but an outstanding manager and *vice versa*),
- how you respond when asked to 'take over', or lead the next session, or in answering the question do you want to manage/lead,
- your view of your actions and the sense you make of what you are trying to achieve and the basis of influence you are drawing on (for example, positional or personal).

These questions, and your responses, are important. They can help you to be clearer about what you want for yourself at work. There is a great difference between being primarily a manager and being primarily a leader in an organization. I have used the word 'primarily' because there will invariably be an element of both, but it is where the emphasis is placed that is the important point to consider.

You need to decide which definition suits you and what you are looking for in the future. These type of questions are rarely considered or analysed in the rush to become a senior professional or role holder. That is not to say that your responses to these questions need not be 'carved in stone', but taking time to ponder on such matters may help you to focus and apply your skills and your efforts more fruitfully over the next few years.

And what about administration? Are leadership and management just different names for *administration*? Will they mean bureaucratic, desk-bound, paperwork-dominated activities? Or is it more the traditional generic term used to describe those who manage? Does being an administrator really mean being a manager or a leader – or both? The only way to decide what a job title means is to find out what the person does. This will tell you if it is more about leadership and/or management.

Characteristics of effective leaders and managers

Put to one side the leadership/management question – I will use the work of Mintzberg (concerning management) and Kouzes and Posner (concerning leadership) to describe those differing roles later in the chapter.

First I want you to consider what you see effective leaders and managers *do* – irrespective of their title. What makes them special and how does their effectiveness manifest itself in practice? Think back to people you know, perhaps with whom you have worked, who were very effective in their leadership or management roles. Make a note of three or four of them from work, your professional training, your social world, school, sports club, etc. What was it that they *did* that had such a positive impact on you and others? The more precise you can be about this the better. Firstly it is valuable for you to recognize what you respect and respond well to, and secondly you can learn from others and adopt their good practices.

Use your responses to build up a framework (see Fig. 11.3) of qualities, which to you constitute effective and productive leadership and managerial behaviours. You can also add in the unhelpful and unproductive things that you see others do. You can then compare and contrast the information to see if it gives you more insights into yourself and how you work. Finally, you can compare your experiences so far with some of the research done by others on the effective practices of leaders and managers. You will then see how your experiences, and you, shape up in relation to their findings in the pages that follow.

Practices of effective leaders – Kouzes and Posner

Please keep the notes you made in Fig. 11.3 in mind as you review what follows.

From their research Kouzes and Posner (1989) have identified a number of attitudes and behaviours common to outstanding leaders. They consider each of us can improve our ability to show these same behaviours and attitudes if we wish to, with adequate training and practice.

They do not subscribe to the view that leaders are born and not made.

(please do this for 2-3 of the people you identified)

1. What did they *do* that made them so successful or influential as a leader or manager?-

    i

    ii

    iii (etc.)

2. What did they *not do* in their role as leader or manager that contributed to their success or influence?

    i

    ii

    iii (etc.)

3. How did you feel as a result of their leadership or managerial behaviour?

    i

    ii

    iii   (etc.)

4. How did they come across in their role to colleagues?

    i

    ii

    iii   (etc.)

Fig. 11.3   Effective leader and manager behaviours: notes from my experience.

They strongly assert that there is nothing mystical or magical about effective leadership: we can all do it if we want to. I believe we each bring with us some natural (genetic) predispositions. I also believe that your hopes for the future are very much in your hands to determine.

Figure 11.4 shows the leadership practices that emerged from the studies of Kouzes and Posner which they present as five *behavioural practices* and ten *commitments*.

Their ideas suggest, that through these practices it is, desirable – and possible – to engage, empower and support one's colleagues to achieve considerable outcomes and to lead them to achieve this for themselves. Each of these specific activities can be taught and assessed to determine

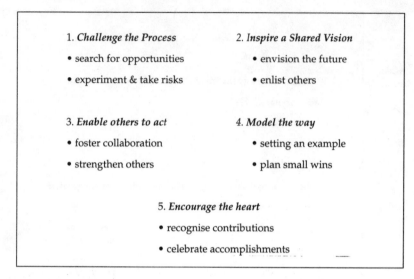

1. *Challenge the Process*

- search for opportunities
- experiment & take risks

2. *Inspire a Shared Vision*

- envision the future
- enlist others

3. *Enable others to act*

- foster collaboration
- strengthen others

4. *Model the way*

- setting an example
- plan small wins

5. *Encourage the heart*

- recognise contributions
- celebrate accomplishments

Fig. 11.4   Practices of exemplary leaders.

the extent to which you consider you currently operate in these ways and where you may need to do more of the practices specified.

Their key message is that outstanding leadership comes from adopting very specific behaviours that can be learnt and practised by each of us. Keep in mind the five main headings in Fig. 11.4 and see to what extent those leaders or managers you rated highly did these things. You can also consider those around you now and assess to what extent these five sets of behaviours appear to be present or absent in your senior colleagues.

Adair and action-centred leadership

John Adair's approach was derived from his work with the military (Adair, 1983). He saw how effective leadership was linked to integrating three interrelated needs:

(1) The needs of the task to be accomplished: clarity about the overall objective together with the actions and behaviours necessary to make it happen.
(2) The needs of the individuals involved: things that help the individual feel a valued part of the team and enable them to make their best contributions.
(3) Attending to group maintenance needs: things that help the group retain its cohesion, its motivation and general willingness to work on the task.

He considers that it is the job of the leader to look at all of these needs at the same time and to keep them in balance as the work proceeds. He depicts these needs as three interlinked circles each of which represents one of the three needs that require attendance (Fig. 11.5).

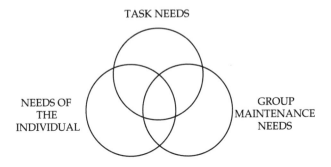

Fig. 11.5 Adair's action-centred leadership.

His framework is simple but powerful and draws attention to the possible consequences of not meeting these three needs sufficiently or of not keeping them in balance. In Fig. 11.6 I have posed three scenarios where one of the three sets of needs is *not* being met. There could be cases where two of the three need clusters are not being met which would lead to major operational difficulties.

What do you think will be the likely consequences for each of these cases set out in Fig. 11.6? What do you think is happening in each of these situations? It may be that you have been in a similar position to one of these, in which case you could draw on your direct experience.

	Task Needs	Individual Needs	Group Needs Maintenance	CONSEQUENCES
Case 1	met	met	not met	? ? ?
Case 2	met	not met	met	? ? ?
Case 3	not met	met	met	? ? ?

Fig. 11.6 Keeping task-individual-the group needs in tune.

Description of scenario	Possible Consequences
Case 1. Group maintenance needs not being met:	Strong emphasis on getting the job done, individual performance matters, little mutual support, possibility of inter-group competition, disintegration of the group possible before the primary task completed, scapegoating etc. etc.
Case 2. Individual needs not being met:	Harmony, collective effort for the common cause emphasised, no space to be an individual, conformity and consensus valued, 'be one of us and do it our way' core messages, could be a build up of rebellion and resistance, feeling of being taken over/smothered etc, etc.
Case 3. Task needs not being met:	Great fun to be in the group where we all support each other and you can be yourself, no attention to getting the core work completed, high risk of being disbanded, could delude itself that it is doing well and no one inside the group would challenge this, etc. etc.

Fig. 11.7   Possible consequences of a needs imbalance.

I have noted in Fig. 11.7 what I would anticipate would be happening in each case.

These are some initial thoughts about how you can use Adair's approach to anticipate problems if these three dimensions are inadequately attended to and balanced in the work of the team, group and meeting. Action centred leadership (ACL) is a well tried and tested approach to developing understanding about leadership. It provides a straightforward way of looking at what is happening. It also focuses the leader's attention on getting the group back on track together.

Situational leadership

This is another very practical approach to management that has appealed to managers. It makes good sense and is not complicated to understand or use. It combines two dimensions that had previously been used to describe different management styles but in this model they are viewed as different dimensions of the same one. These are:

- the extent to which the leader *directs the tasks* to be done,
- the emphasis given to building a *supportive relationship* with staff.

Rather than looking at these as either/or styles of leadership, research studies at Ohio State University suggested that much of leader behaviour could be classified into task and relationship initiated behaviour. Also, far from these dimensions being seen as competing theories of leadership they existed together. This led to a two-dimensional theory of leadership and an approach that was eventually called 'situational leadership' developed by Hersey and Blanchard (1988).

The model suggests that – as the leader – you always need to give your staff some *direction* about the work to be done, and you also need to build up your work *relationship* with them to support them in their work. The amount of attention you give to each of these two dimensions varies depending on the competence each person has for the specific jobs undertaken.

So, you need to manage each person differently, because of personality differences, and also depending on the particular job they are doing, because they can be extremely competent and experienced at certain aspects of their job but less experienced with others. What they are saying is that there is no one best way of managing, or of being a leader. You need to match your style to the needs of the person you are managing at all times, hence the term of *situational* leadership, and from task to task.

By putting the concern for task, and the concern for relationship dimensions together, Hersey and Blanchard came up with the framework in Fig. 11.8. This one is the result of work done by Paul Hersey but developed from their earlier work together. It shows four styles depending on the balance given to directive and relationship leadership.

There is a developmental sequence of leadership style which goes from:

- *Telling:* making sure that the person knows what is to be done, and receives the direction needed while they learn the necessary skills etc., then the leader's style can move to
- *Selling:* when the leader is still in charge but is engaging more of the interest of the staff person; from this stage the impetus moves from the leader.

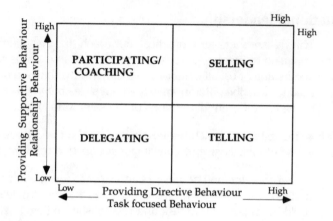

Fig. 11.8 The Situational leadership framework.

- *Participating and coaching:* at this stage the primary responsibility for action has transferred over to the employee who requires more of a coaching role and the leader puts less effort into directing because he now has a more experienced member of staff.
- *Delegating:* is adopted by the leader when he recognizes the competence of his staff to be fully responsible for the work to be done, and that the best thing he can do is let his member of staff get on with the job, while still offering support.

Remember that the leadership style you adopt should be related to that person doing a specific part of their work. It is probably inaccurate to assume that just because they need a lot of instruction and direction for task 'A' they need the same for task 'B'. Even if you recruited a very experienced nurse specialist you will need to adopt a 'telling' style during their initial introductory period. They need time to settle into their new surroundings and find out how things are done in the new setting. Help them adjust and get to grips with the local procedures. Then you will be able to let go and manage them through a delegative style more quickly than if you just pushed them in at the deep end to cope alone.

The model is very flexible and reflects how each of us can be very competent at one part of our job but less so about others. I know from personal experience how worrying it can be when it is assumed, because you can do certain things, that you will be able to do different, but related, tasks you have not come across before with no real guidance. In such a situation just a little bit of 'telling' can give you the direction and security you need to perform your tasks. You can then rapidly move through to being managed in a 'delegating' style when appropriate.

These models are very interesting and practical and I hope they have sparked an interest in you to find out more. There are references and further reading at the end of the chapter for you to follow up more extensively. There are questionnaires available, for Kouzes and Posner (1989) and for situational leadership. These will help you identify your current styles of working and identify where you may be able to enhance your performance through using different styles to those you currently rely on.

Mintzberg: the nature of managerial work

These ideas were derived from observing what managers actually did as opposed to what they said they did. Mintzberg (1980) found that the manager's day was very hectic. There was little – if any – time for long periods of reflection and most of the time he or she was dealing with people either face to face or on the phone at a very hectic pace.

He systematically looked at what managers did, the characteristics of their jobs and how they were set up to function in their different organizations. He asked managers to keep detailed diaries, and he – and his colleagues – followed them around. They talked about their day to day work in great detail. The following ten key roles of a manager emerged from the field work; they are organized into three role clusters as shown in Fig. 11.9.

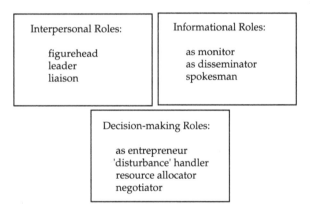

Fig. 11.9 Ten roles of a manager.

He found that managers move between these ten key roles throughout the day. Figure 11.10 indicates how these ten key roles relate to the different types of managerial work a person has to do to remain effective.

If you run through these two lists – depending on your experience – which of these roles have you experienced so far? At first glance some of them may not seem to be relevant to health care. But remembering

Managerial Job Type	Key Roles
Contact man	liaison, figurehead
Political manager	spokesman, negotiator
Entrepreneur	entrepreneur, negotiator
Insider	resource allocator
Real-time manager	disturbance-handler
Team manager	leader
Expert manager	monitor, spokesman
New manager	liaison, monitor

Fig. 11.10 Relating managerial types to key managerial roles.

the changes and the creation of the internal market, some of these roles, primarily drawn from the world of commercial business, will increasingly apply to aspects of the managerial roles we see in health. You may like to make a note in Fig. 11.11 of the job types and roles that interest you. This could also set you thinking about new directions for your career.

Managerial Job Type		Key Roles	
Experienced	Interested by ...	Experienced	Interested by...
•	•	•	•
•	•	•	•
•	•	•	•
•	•	•	•

Fig. 11.11 Noting my experience and interest in Mintzberg's roles.

Mintzberg (1980) has upset some of his academic colleagues by concentrating on what managers *actually* do rather than suggesting high-level ideas about what top managers *should* do. However he has removed some of the mystique about management and brought this type of work down to earth.

When you look at Mintzberg's work ask yourself two simple questions:

(1)   Do I want to be doing this sort of work later in my career?
(2)   Am I capable of such work later in my career?

Depending on your answers you have something to go on to guide your efforts and shape your aspirations for the next few years.

It could be that your views about managers, and how people are motivated, have been shaped by other influences. These may include some influential ideas from Douglas McGregor (1960), an American social psychologist.

McGregor's theory X and theory Y

This is perhaps the most well known of all the theories of management and motivation. Through his work the contrast between strongly opposing views about the nature of people in work has been most starkly portrayed. He proposed, and contrasted, two very different philosophies of man. Each had major implications for defining what management was seen to be about and how management should motivate their staff. I believe his model continues to exercise a major influence on much of current everyday thinking about business management. You thus need to be familiar with his ideas, even if you disagree with some of the points he makes.

He proposed two contrasting propositions about people at work:

(1)   workers have to be *directed and controlled* (the notion of theory X),
(2)   workers are intrinsically *self-motivating and self-directed* (the notion of theory Y).

These theories have become deeply embedded concepts of management thinking and influence our approach to:

- performance management
- appraisal
- staff development
- reward strategies
- work process re-organization
- motivation at work
- successful management practice.

The characteristics of the two work philosophies are as follows:

The assumptions of theory X:

- The average human being has an inherent dislike of work and will avoid it if he can.
- Due to this dislike of work, most people must be coerced, controlled, directed or threatened with punishment to get them to put forth adequate effort toward the achievement of organizational objectives.
- The average person prefers to be directed, wishes to avoid responsibility, has relatively little ambition and, above all, wants security.

This theory is essentially pessimistic and restrictive in the view of man that is presented. Man has to be pushed, cajoled and directed to do what needs to be done. You have to watch them all the time otherwise they may be slipshod and if you look away they will avoid doing the job. You cannot trust them: they have no inherent interest in the job and they just want the money and watch the clock until it is time to go home. It reduces everyone to the lowest common denominator. Little acknowledgement is given to those who don't fit this picture, who would probably be viewed as trying to hoodwink the management in some way and 'need to be watched!'.

The assumptions of theory Y:

- The expenditure of physical and mental effort in work is as natural as play or rest.
- External control and the threat of punishment are not the only means for bringing about effort toward organizational objectives.
- Man will exercise self-direction and self-control in the service of objectives to which he is committed.
- Commitment to objectives is a function of the rewards associated with their achievement.
- The average person learns, under proper conditions, not only to accept but to seek responsibility.
- The capacity to exercise a relatively high degree of imagination, ingenuity and creativity in the solution of organizational problems is widely, not narrowly, distributed in the population.
- Under the conditions of modern industrial life, the intellectual potentialities of the human being are only partially utilized.

These assumptions have sharply different implications for managerial strategy than do those of theory X. They are dynamic rather than static. They acknowledge the possibility for individual growth and development. They allow for several ways of engaging with and motivating people rather than a single absolute form of directive control. Theory Y proposes a more creative and optimistic vision of man and his potential.

Theory X offers management an easy rationalization for ineffective organization performance. It suggests that it is due to the nature of the human resources (which are inherently untrustworthy) with which we must work. Theory Y, on the other hand, places operational problems squarely in the lap of management who had not been able to bring out the necessary skills and abilities needed.

The descriptions summarized for theories X and Y are a bit extreme but they do indicate two very different systems of belief about the nature of work, the purpose of management, and the nature of man. You may like to reflect on your philosophy of management, and also that of your managers and colleagues. Think about theory X and theory Y; where would you place yourself on a scale of 1–10 (see Fig. 11.12)?

		Preference for Theories X & Y
		1 (low) ---- 5 ---- 10(high)
My philosophy of management	Theory X	
	Theory Y	
Colleagues' philosophy	Theory X	
	Theory Y	
My Managers' philosophy	Theory X	
	Theory Y	
The Organisation's philosophy	Theory X	
	Theory Y	

Fig. 11.12 Reflections on the accuracy of theory x and theory Y.

At best these will be your impressions of what may be guiding the thinking behind management decisions where you work. The results may shock you as there may be a difference between what people say they believe in and what they actually do in practice. Look out for such discrepancies as they relate back to some of the material discussed in Chapter 3 on organizations.

McGregor considered that behind every managerial decision or action there were assumptions about human nature and human behaviour. Revealing these could do much to illuminate the styles of individual managers and how the organization itself operates. These insights could facilitate a rich and constructive review of what we expect from others and thus one of the bases on which we make our expectations.

Conclusion

A great deal of material has been introduced in Part Three with the intention of providing different ways to reconsider the practices and processes that are in operation where you work. While Part Two kept the focus on you as a person, Part Three focused on your operational relationships at work and the many dimensions which require attention.

Part Three was not intended to convince you of any one particular approach to follow. It suggested you query the many things going on around you, not all of which are conscious, and pay more attention to the dynamics involved in providing health care. It also suggested you open up several different avenues of thought and decide which ones make most sense for you to follow.

However, knowing about more things and generally being more aware is not of any use if you cannot make the changes required. Facilitating change in organizations is very difficult to achieve, but that is the focus for Part Four. It builds directly on the material of the first three parts and will set out several tried and tested approaches that you can use, when appropriate, to help constructive change happen.

References

Adair, J. (1983) *Effective Leadership*, Gower Publishing, Aldershot.

Hersey, P. and Blanchard, K. (1988) *Management of Human Resources*, Prentice-Hall, Englewood Cliffs, NJ.

Kotter, J. (1982) *The General Manager*, Free Press, New York.

Kouzes, J. and Posner, B. (1989) *The Leadership Challenge*, Jossey-Bass, San Francisco.

McGregor, D. (1960) *The Human Side of Enterprise* McGraw-Hill, New York.

Mintzberg, H. (1980) *The Nature of Managerial Work*, Prentice-Hall, Englewood Cliffs, NJ.

Further reading

Ackoff, R. (1986) *Management in Small Doses*, Wiley, New York.

Bennis, W. and Nanus, B. (1985) *Leaders*, Harper and Row, New York.

Bowman, M. (1986) *Nursing Management*, Croom Helm, Beckenham.

Clutterbuck, D. and Crainer, S. (1990) *Makers of Management*, MacMillan, London.

Fulghum, R. (1990) *All I Need to Know I Learned in Kindergarten*, Grafton Books, London.

Handy, C. (1990) *Inside Organizations*, BBC Books, London.

Harvey-Jones, J. (1990) *Trouble Shooter*, BBC Books, London.

Heider, J. (1986) *The Tao of Leadership*, Gower, Aldershot.

Levinson, H. and Rosenthal, S. (1984) *CEO Corporate Leadership in Action*, Basic Books, New York.

O'Leary, J. *et al.* (1986) *Winning Strategies for Nursing Managers*, JB Lippincott Co, Philadelphia.

McKenna, E. (1994) *Business Psychology* and *Organisational Behaviour*, Lawrence Erlbaum Associates Ltd, Hove.

Morgan, G. (1993) *Imaginization: The Art of Creative Management*. Sage, London.

Peters, T. and Waterman, R. (1982) *In Search of Excellence*, Harper and Row, New York.

Quick, T. (1985) *The Manager's Motivation Desk Book*, Wiley, New York.

Stewart, R. (1982) *Choices for the Manager*, McGraw-Hill, Maidenhead.

Stewart, R. (1989) *Leading in the NHS*, Macmillan, Basingstoke.

Torrington, D., Weightman, J. and Johns, K. (1989) *Effective Management*, Prentice-Hall, Hemel Hempstead.

Vaill, P. (1989) *Managing as a Performing Art*, Jossey-Bass, San Francisco.

Video Arts (1984) *So You Think You Can Manage?* Methuen, London.

PART FOUR:
CHANGE AND CHANGING

Part Four sets out some practical ways of thinking about the dynamics of change, and considers the role of the nurse as a force for change. It is not possible to 'manage change' in a detailed and predictable way yet the processes of change can be guided and shaped to a considerable extent. These chapters (i) explore the inherent difficulties involved in facilitating change, (ii) set out several sound and well-tried ways of preparing for, and shaping, the processes of change, and (iii) look at the nurse as a 'change-agent'.

If I asked 100 people to describe the role and activities of a nurse, the overwhelming response I suspect would concentrate on the caring or curative aspects of your work. I suspect very few would mention the role of the nurse in helping patients cope with change and adapt to a new situation. Yet this is a core component of a nurse's role. All the time you are involved in facilitating patients' adaptation to their changing clinical and social conditions; changes in their attitude to their life ahead; changes to new and different treatment regimes; and changes in ward practice and management. I see the role of the nurse in facilitating personal, group and organizational change as significant but often unrecognized.

So much of the day-to-day running of clinics and hospitals revolves around the operational decisions made by nurses. How they choose to interpret and then act on the decisions received from more senior colleagues can dramatically affect the whole tone and feel of a ward, department, or clinic. This aspect of every nurse's role and responsibility may not be sufficiently emphasized or given very much attention.

Chapter 12
Why is Organizational Change so Difficult?

Making changes actually happen is a neglected field of study. Much attention is given to theorizing about 'the management of change' and on diagnosis but relatively little attention is given to focusing on the things that get in the way of the planned changes actually occurring! Part of this comes from approaching the processes of change as if they were logical or rational ones, and capable of being predicted and ordered to a level which is not possible.

Deciding what needs to change, and why, is very important. Yet, too often it appears as if the taking of a decision to change is the really difficult part. Making the change happen seems to demand less attention. We know from experience that it is not quite that simple. The problems invariably encountered often lead to increasing pressure for change being applied – through more facts and figures, or perhaps through putting pressure on those resisting the proposals – response.

There is a belief that if people see the rational case for a change they will be impelled to make the changes so clearly described. Nothing could be further from the truth. Certainly the logic, formal data and the rationality of a change proposal are very influential, but they are not the only matters to look at in enabling change to happen.

This chapter looks at some of the reasons why blocks and barriers stop and frustrate the implementation of change in organizations; change which is appropriate, soundly based, and needed. The problem is that each of us always see things from *our* own perspective. Sometimes we see things very differently, not because of logic but because of personal difference.

This adds to the complexity of performing a logical and rational appraisal of the change needed. Account must also be taken of the impact of such planned changes on the people directly affected by them.

The complexity of organizational change

Since the 1970s, the NHS has been in almost continuous flux and subject to imposed external structural changes that altered:

- its managerial infrastructure very substantially,
- introduced a competitive internal market,
- put to the test – some would say breaking point – the philosophy of health care delivery based on clinical need rather than resource availability.

All this adds up to institutional change on a massive scale. This was propelled through the NHS by the weight of the government departments and regional structure and underpinned by considerable thought and planning.

Yet not all the imposed changes have gone according to plan and there continue to be casualties. People choose to resist or speak 'out of turn', and the stress and strain of trying to make the imposed changes happen continues to affect many. There is also a huge difference between designing a large-scale change and its practical implementation. Difficulties may not always be recognized by the planners and shapers of institutional change.

Why should this be? The objective rationality of, for example, 'Care in the Community' and the introduction of a general management ethos (The Griffiths Report, 1983) are understandable in themselves and make 'sense'. Yet they were resisted, reinterpreted, resented and repelled by many. In return they were reiterated, imposed and forced into a, largely unwilling, service. Yet the notions and their intention on which they are based have merit.

What is the problem? Is it new ideas *per se*, or trying to adapt to new ideas? Is it about letting go of what you know, or about loss of power? The list could go on and on. There are many matters to take into account when considering changing the *status quo*. Yet the approach usually followed only emphasizes the logic and the rational case for the proposed changes. To my mind this is only part of the story. It is quite inadequate on its own when moving towards implementation.

It is difficult to generate change along the lines you want in an organization. Causing some disruption to the *status quo* is not in itself difficult at all. The challenge is in containing the anxiety you create when you make a change *and* in nudging and shaping it towards the outcomes you want to achieve. Recall how cautious and resistant you can be when asked to embrace something new. This will remind you of how difficult coping with change can be. If you then multiply this many times it gives a clue to the complexity of facilitating change within an organization. To do this across the health service, for example, shows how difficult it is to plan, control, contain and achieve.

The position is complicated further because the architects of change are rarely the implementors of the proposed plans and ideas. There often appears to be a big gap between how change is talked about in the abstract (very tidy and neat) and how it is in practice (messy, confusing and problematic). Sometimes the problems arise because change is discussed as if the organization (department, team, function, location, etc.) was a passive entity that will embrace the new changes 'just like that'. There can be a misplaced optimism, an arrogance at times, by the instigators of change in organizations that they appear to know what the problems are and, therefore, what needs to be done. This can lead them to ignore the wisdom and experience of those in the field.

Several years ago I was working with a board (not in health care) who were trying to manage the effects of their collapsing market. In many ways they had become too complacent and tried to manage things from a distance rather than getting back into the market to find out what it was like 'in the front line' as it were. I started asking what sort of generals they were like. After some confusion we began discussing the difference between 'armchair generals' (the board) and field-based generals (which was what they needed to become!). It had quite a shocking impact. While the board wanted the company to do well and had immense intellectual capabilities, they had lost contact with their staff and their markets. Therefore they had problems with the new conditions surrounding them.

The introduction of a change triggers testing and checking-out responses from those affected by it which are intended to clarify what the proposed change is about, the effect it will have on current practice, job security, seniority, career development etc. While a viable and necessary alternative to current practice is proposed, it may be seen by others as a challenging and unnecessary indictment of their past performance and future capability. This is especially so if they consider they will be worse off than before. It can generate resistance and anxiety.

In every situation we bring our own bias, past experience and intuitive assessments to bear. In an organization and in groups these checking processes become even more complicated and difficult to work with. We get phenomena occurring, such as 'Group think' (Janis, 1972) and the Abilene Paradox (Harvey, 1988). Also there are examples of a phenomena known as 'risky-shift' (Wallach *et al*, 1968). When working in a group, this is where the decisions taken can become more risky and questionable than a member's individual assessment and decision making would be. This suggests that in group settings the combination of the collective experiences and knowledge can lead to less soundly based outcomes than if individuals responded on their own judgement alone. The culture of the group, and the culture of the organization, influences an individual's assessment of a situation and their judgement.

Another determining factor affecting the quality of the decisions made is the emotional potency of the group at the time of reaching a decision, and the criticality of the issues under consideration. What is clear is that the process of change in individuals and for organizations is *not* a rational or logical process alone; other influential processes come into play.

In summary:

- Logical, rational initiatives will often be resisted if they mean change to the current arrangements.
- True views and feelings are not always expressed.
- In collective settings collective wisdom can result in collective foolishness.
- After the event we are not always clear about why we acted as we did.
- Change means disruption to many and implies a criticism of their past performance.

Organizational change is a mixed up and complicated affair because of the implications it holds about personal security, competence and meaning. This is due to the anxiety it raises for those affected by the proposals being made. No matter how careful, bright and far-sighted the instigators of change may be, unless they tap into these non-organizational facets of change their best efforts can be frustrated, misconstrued and resisted.

What *is* going on around me?

Much is written about how an organization is there to meet its mission or its core purpose. This is usually defined by varying statements of objectives and achievements. What is not often stated is how organizations also exist to meet and satisfy the individual and collective needs of those who work there. Usually these needs are met by individual members doing (or resisting) their formal work 'in their own way'. It is also achieved through the informal organization that operates alongside the formal hierarchy.

Organizations seek not only to achieve their formally stated business goals, but also to respond to the collective dynamics of their members. Recognizing this introduces another way of looking at how each of us relates to and behaves within our organization. This *personal–dynamic* dimension influences individual and collective thinking and behaviour. For some the organization represents their main purpose in life. For others the organization offers a means of defending themselves against life's uncertainties and traumas. In different ways members of an organization psychologically invest parts of themselves in that organization and they have a strong and vested interest in any attempts to alter the *status quo*. It is not surprising therefore that change will not be simple to achieve. This is especially so if that change undermines an aspect of my personal life security.

Organizations not only bring people together to accomplish predetermined tasks (e.g. provide health services), they are also intensely socially-dynamic entities that function on several levels of interaction. In health care this complexity is increased because of the changing population of patients and relatives. What is already a complicated entity (the organization) becomes increasingly so.

This suggests that what goes on in an organization cannot be fully understood by just applying conventional business concepts. Within an organization there is an important emotional attachment, which can be both positive and negative. It is felt by those within it and transforms the organization from a set of connected boxes on an organization chart to that of an intensely emotional and dynamic workplace.

The emotional dynamics within organizations are not unusual features nor should they be unexpected. However, because they are not usually talked about, they remain difficult and uncomfortable matters to consider openly. It is far easier to talk instead about performance figures and plans for the future. What would be constructive would be to categorize, and thus legitimize for more consideration, the emotional dynamics. Also to then observe the effect they may have on group performance. Being more aware and encouraged to consider these aspects of organizational life could enhance both the individual and the organization's ability to cope with change.

One way of differentiating between the different levels of an organization's dynamics is by contrasting the extent to which there is open and freely shared knowledge about the interactions taking place. Figure 12.1 suggests that there are three levels of interactions at play: the manifest, the covert and the unconscious.

The 'first level' is that of manifest behaviour covering what is said out

Level of Dynamics	The Type of Influence	Description of the behaviour
First Level What is there for all to see	Explicit intentions Implicit intentions (access is open to all)	MANIFEST BEHAVIOUR
Second Level What is there for only some to see	Covert intentions (access is hidden, restricted to the selected few)	COVERT BEHAVIOUR
Third Level What is there but not consciously seen by any	Psycho-dynamic and unconscious intentions, drives and tensions	UNCONSCIOUS COMMUNICATIONS

Fig. 12.1 Three levels of organizational dynamics.

loud and what is implied. The 'second level' is where some information is only known by some of the group and is purposefully not shared. Here there is the potential for duplicitous activity, misinformation or covert actions. The 'third level' of unconscious, and not known, forces and dynamics exert an influence on organizational behaviour.

Nearly all of my initial professional training emphasized the level one interactions and dynamics. Often there was a strong adverse reaction to any suggestions of the covert ways of working that occur in organizations. But it is the third level that from my experience is invariably denied, or laughed off as not existing. I suspect there is much that occurs beneath the surface that influences what we do, see, feel and hear at work.

The problem is that since these influences are out of awareness, we cannot readily describe, define or capture them in any direct way. We can look for them in disguised and derivative forms though, and wonder what may be going on from these glimpses of the unconscious. One consequence of discounting the impact of such 'out-of-awareness' influences is that it puts more pressure on us to account for unreasonable or bizarre behaviour which is out of context for the person or group concerned. We even try to give logical explanations for it. If we acknowledge the possibility of level three influences, it could open up a new way of thinking about our behaviour at work. It would also help to make more sense of unusual, bizarre or unexpected behaviour.

One of the reasons why working in organized settings can become so difficult is because we focus on the procedural, mechanistic and operational aspects of work. We are directed to forget, deny, postpone, put aside or to diminish the 'human' side of work. Yet it is through relationships, collaborations, rivalries etc., that the formal business problems are resolved. By denying the irrational (or at least the other than logical – rational) side of us we miss an important part of the total picture.

Sorting out the procedures, monitoring performance etc., is important in providing efficient health care but it is not the whole story. The relative denial of ourselves in organizations can lead to staff being seen as just another set of resources to be managed and controlled. It also leads to a view, or expectation, that organizations can be set up and will function according to a logical and rational assessment of the hard facts. The experience of working in an organization does not fully bear out these expectations.

The dynamics of disruption: management of change?

Given the presence of such strong psychological attachments it should come as no surprise that changing an organization is difficult to achieve. This is particularly so if attention is only given to the organization's formal business agenda.

Change in an organization generates considerable anxiety and a fear of loss of what is known. Consequently, attempts at change are likely to be experienced as destabilizing factors. This will create resistance. Attempts at change *will* involve a restructuring of the embedded patterns of organizational attitudes and relationships. Unless this whole framework of issues, dynamics and considerations is taken into account the attempt to change is likely to be persistently resisted.

What is often insufficiently acknowledged, or addressed, is that at the heart of successful organizational change is the taking of many individual decisions to re-commit to the new situation. Unless this can be achieved with the staff affected it is unlikely that changes introduced will be successful or maintained. This is one of the reasons why successful change in organizations is so difficult to accomplish.

The anxiety generated during times of organizational upheaval is seen by Levinson (1970) to contain four types of loss:

- the loss of love
- the loss of support
- the loss of sensory input
- the loss of the capacity to act.

He sees the sense of loss experienced (e.g. during a merger – say between two units, or the formation of a health commission from two previously separate ones) as touching people very deeply. It is something which, unless handled with great care and sensitivity, undermines our capacity to trust. You may recall from Part Two that trust was at the core of Erik Erikson's psycho-social model of human development (Erikson, 1982). Erikson saw this as the basic strength that underlied all other psychological strengths.

This notion has been applied by Gilkey (1991) to merger activities who observes how

> In failing to re-establish employees' capacities for basic trust, autonomy and initiative these ventures frequently flounder. They are unable to overcome the regressive impact of such major reorganisation and restore the strengths and commitments of their employees . . .

Gilkey notes how mergers and acquisitions often fail because inadequate attention is given to recognizing, understanding and managing the psychological factors involved in such engagements. 'Mergers and acquisitions, like any major change, disrupt individual and organisational equilibrium. Old psychological contracts are broken, loyalties and informal networks are undermined, and the earlier sense of purpose and direction is often lost.' At this time of continuing change it could be that these insights should be applied to NHS merger activity.

Erikson's model can be used to chart and anticipate some of the likely concerns of those in the midst of imposed change. It could also be used as a basis for planning the management of change in addition to the more formalized business approaches conventionally applied.

Why haven't these ideas been taken up more fully?

Since the turn of the century the insights triggered by Freud's initial writings (Freud, 1900) about the unconscious have suggested that unseen psychological forces exert a major influence on what we think, believe and do. Elton Mayo achieved some ground-breaking social psychological research (Mayo, 1945) into work group behaviour. He and others have documented that the motivation and behaviour of employees is not solely driven by instrumental task accomplishment but by other, primarily social, influences. From both the individual psycho-analytical world, and from the world of work psychology there has been recognition of the presence and significant effect that other than logical or 'seen' influences have on individual and collective action.

More recognition is now given to the possibility that behaviour in organizations can be distorted by unconscious or out-of-awareness processes – as with individuals – and from psychological anxieties generated by work settings. This highlights the possibility that so-called logical decision making and effective management practice may be influenced by additional, other-than-rational drives and processes; drives and processes that are elusive to define and hard to pin down.

The clinical premise of not taking for granted what is directly observable can be applied to organizations too. You may like to look beyond the obvious behaviours, and practices and consider if part of what you see and experience is in response to an organization's more hidden and deeper motives and needs.

It is surprising that, in spite of growing acknowledgement of their importance, socio-psycho-dynamic insights on organizations and groups have not been used more frequently. Some reasons for this are set out in Fig. 12.2 below and it may be that until these are confronted many of the insights available to help you in your work will continue to be missed, misinterpreted or denied.

These possible barriers suggest that there is a tension and a nervousness about exploring the impact of unconscious internal processes on the behaviour of organizations. If these suppositions are accurate this may be because:

- there is insufficient awareness of what this would mean in practice,
- it would bring to the surface unacceptable material,
- it would be too difficult to handle and work with at a personal level,
- to do so is not seen as a legitimate part of the manager's role.

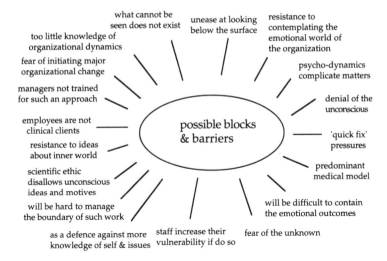

Fig. 12.2 Possible blocks and barriers to working with the dynamics of the organization.

It may be that to achieve a 'good enough' balance between the demands of the organization and the psychological needs of their employees, organizations will have to search for ways of legitimizing, and integrating, the business and the individual needs of its work force. In this way a vastly neglected side of organizational life could be acknowledged and validated as important. Its impact on facilitating, and understanding, the processes of individual and organizational change is huge.

More attention should be paid to people's experiences in organizations. By using these perceptives we will realize that we are all subject to the same anxieties, compulsions and dilemmas as everyone else. No matter how compelling our logical arguments about an issue may be, we will have to acknowledge our own unconscious desires and defences. This is regardless of whether we are the chief executive, a clinical director, a senior nurse manager or the most junior nurse in training. This may be uncomfortable to acknowledge and accept.

If change stimulates such a complex set of reactions then it needs to be approached with a degree of seriousness and sophistication that is not always apparent as far as the dynamic aspects are concerned. Change initiatives should be thought through and planned as far as possible taking more account of the psychological attachments staff form with their work groups and their organization as a whole. This is because change affects staff at a deeply personal level.

Change in organizations is not a matter of working out great ideas on paper and expecting these will then be readily transferred into practice. The reality is that change will be confusing for many. It will be messy and there is a likelihood of unexpected and unwanted fallout. It will also take time, often far longer than expected. The ideas on paper will *not* work out precisely as planned in practice. People will be anxious; blocks, barriers, misinformation will occur, etc.

Change is not a neutral business; there is invariably pain and trauma, suffering and delight. All these reactions and responses need to be acknowledged and addressed if the process and the outcomes are to be worthwhile and effective. What can be done to anticipate some of these considerations is to acknowledge some of the concerns and tensions and try to address them with those affected.

In Chapter 13 we consider some ideas and ways of structuring the change process. In Chapter 14 we consider the role of the nurse as a sponsor, as a facilitator and as a 'change agent'.

References

Erikson, E. (1982) *The Life Cycle Completed*, WW Norton, New York.

Freud, S. (1900) *The Interpretation of Dreams*, Standard Edition, Hogarth Press, London.

Gilkey, R. (1991) The psychodynamics of upheaval, in Kets de Vries (ed.) *Organizations on the Couch*, Jossey-Bass, San Francisco.

Harvey, J. (1988) *The Abilene Paradox*, Lexington Books, Lexington, MA.

Janis, J. (1972) *Victims of Groupthink*, Houghton Mifflin Co, Boston, MA.

Levinson, H. (1970) A psychologist diagnoses merger failures. *Harvard Business Review*, **48**, 2.

Mayo, E. (1945) *The Social Problems of an Industrial Civilization*, Harvard University Press.

NHS Management Inquiry (1983) The Griffiths Report, DHSS, London.

Wallach, M. *et al.* (1968) Group influence on individual risk-taking, in D. Cartwright and A. Zander *Group Dynamics: Research and Theory*, Harper and Row, London.

Chapter 13
Planning for Change

Since much has been written about 'the management of change' my aim is to outline some of the essential ideas and keep this chapter brief. I don't believe it is possible to manage change as such because there are too many variables occurring at the same time and just when you think you have everything sorted you can turn round and slip on the proverbial banana skin. However there are many actions you can take which reduce the tensions, confusions and uncertainties associated with change. But I don't think we can ever manage change in the sense of having everything neatly planned and sorted. Nor can you predict precisely how the planned changes will work out in practice.

However being able to reduce some of the inherent instability and personal anxiety triggered by changing situations is reassuring. It gives you back the ability to cope with the course of events and to influence their outcomes.

Why is *change* so difficult?

Every day we have to respond to the changing situations in which we find ourselves. So much of our existence requires us to respond to change that it could be said that consequently we should be very accomplished and practised in the art of coping with change. It may be a surprise to describe life in this way and then as a shock to acknowledge that, in spite of our lifetime of practice, we continue to experience problems in coping with change!

It can be a burden to constantly cope with change. We never seem to have any choice. Thus one of the ways in which we can cope is to emphasize the formal patterns around which we structure our lives.

Work is very important in helping us structure and order the changing world. It provides us with boundaries to use as a basis for organizing our life and for defining our relationships with others. The formalized ways we follow in going about business give us a measure of regularity and predictability. However this really is an illusion, because everything is in a state of movement.

The end result is that each of us is guided, even dominated, by a routinization of life that are productive for us for much of the time. We can create expected and realistic patterns of behaviour and establish mutual expectations with others. This provides us with an acceptable measure of continuity that allows us to keep our life in order.

If we are to help change in organizations to take place, in ways that do not leave people feeling violated, ignored, dispossessed etc., we need to take into account the concerns they have when the possibility of change is raised. We need to remember the possibility that the rules and procedures they follow have an additional psychological purpose of creating the impression of permanence and order.

Following routines and procedures gives a sense of security and continuity. When these are put at risk – as when changes are proposed – far more than a procedural change, or a reporting relationship is involved.

Figure 13.1 notes some of the reasons why change is resisted. Drawing on your experience, add in more reasons. If you are more aware of what gets in the way of necessary constructive change, for you and for others, then you can take such worries and concerns into account in the planning and consultation process.

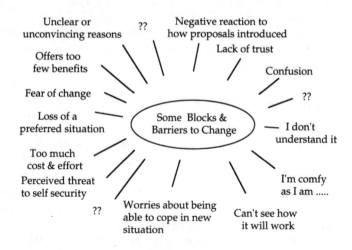

Fig. 13.1   Some barriers to change.

The responses noted above give a clue about how to address each of these reactions. The person initiating the changes just needs to take them on board. For example, if those affected don't understand what is being proposed, or perhaps have fears about job security, then one immediate remedy is to acknowledge the concerns expressed. Then either explain more carefully what is being proposed and/or discuss job security. The key is to try to understand what the issues are, no matter how trivial or 'silly' they may appear to be on the surface. Then address them with respect and due care.

If the people affected are under stress or worried then more attention is needed to explain and work through the issues. You may have a patient who is to be transferred or where their treatment is to be changed. The issue could be the breaking up of a training set after being together for a couple of years or a move you need to make, for training purposes, to a different speciality. Whatever the case, each needs to be discussed and worked through sufficiently if the change is to have a reasonable chance of being successful.

In order to help others and yourself cope with change, you could consider what the proposed changes would mean if you were in their place. This will give you an insight into how others look at matters and why they are responding as they do. Effective change is about a person making a decision to work with new arrangements with belief and positive purpose. Sometimes there is no choice but to go along with proposals for change. However, the potential for pent-up anger, a sense of being 'done to' and a preparedness to sabotage the changes will persist unless their internal frustration and tension is addressed.

A key to resolving barriers to change is to ask yourself the question 'What do I need to do or think about, that will help each person affected make the changes needed?' There will be colleagues who will resist the changes to be made. However, by at least appreciating their opposition and taking their reservations into account you can acknowledge their right to protest even if the changes still proceed. It is rarely possible to meet the needs of everyone. It *is* possible to hear what everyone wants and needs to say and to consider their views.

If I am to promote a change at work, or if I am to be affected by a change imposed on me, these are some of the conditions I need to have met. Also these are some of the questions I need answered, or to answer:

Understanding why the change is needed

- opportunity to challenge and test the proposals,
- clarity of what I can/cannot influence,
- opportunity to contribute if desired,
- awareness of the personal consequences for me,
- awareness of impact on others,
- understanding why the *status quo* cannot remain,
- What are benefits and losses of the change.

Looking to the future

- consider the possibilities,
- building up a picture of what it could be like,

- what is the best and worst scenarios,
- how long will things take,
- what is the prognosis.

Knowing what to do

- what is to be required of me,
- when will some changes start,
- who is to do what, and to whom,
- what is the project plan,
- what are the immediate next steps.

What other questions would you want to answer in addition to these?

Planning the change process

Having set the scene, the rest of this chapter (i) introduces a framework for initiating changes and (ii) introduces some practical models for diagnosing your situation before initiating the change process are then introduced. You can use these ideas to help prepare for and then initiate a change process. You can also use them to diagnose what is going on in your organization, or elsewhere.

A framework for review

There are a series of steps you need to take to plan any change. First you need to decide if change is required. Second, discovering if change is a viable and realistic option. Both of these conditions need to be met. To push for change when the organization cannot sustain it is foolhardy. To make change when it is not needed is exploitative and somewhat narcissistic. You require both the need for change and the capability within the organization for it to be achievable.

If one of these is not present – leave things as they are for the time being. If there is a need for change but you don't believe that the organization can cope with it, you will need to build up the organization's internal capability. This includes such areas as skills, systems, experience etc to a point where the changes needed can be initiated.

When you have reached a position where it is practical and viable to go ahead, you must think through the change process before taking action. One approach could be to use a framework like the one depicted in Fig. 13.2 to structure your preparatory thinking. Not only does it help you build up a more complete picture of your situation but it forces you to sketch out an action plan and to consider how to maintain the changed arrangements once they have been introduced.

This planning framework consists of five stages each of which requires attention. Successful change is not only about diagnosing the need for change, deciding what is needed and doing it as quickly as possible. Considerable attention also needs to be given to how the process can best be handled. What support for the staff affected will be provided? What arrangements will be put in place to help the new arrangements be sustained after the major changes have been made?

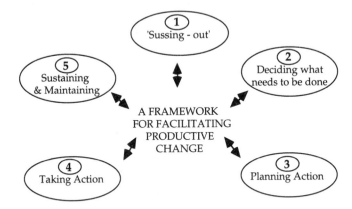

Fig. 13.2 A planning framework for productive change.

Figure 13.2 shows the five main stages located around the purpose of the framework to facilitate productive and sustainable change. Each of these stages is briefly outlined below.

(1) Investigating the current situation (intervening to find out)
  (a) what is the current position,
  (b) where am I in it all,
  (c) historical background,
  (d) emergent issues and problems,
  (e) any 'emergency' conditions to attend to.
(2) Deciding what needs to be done (diagnosing the issues and opportunities)
  (a) describing the initial business diagnosis,
  (b) setting out the problems and alternative solutions,
  (c) assessing what is ethical, viable and practical to do,
  (d) anticipating problems and difficulties,
  (e) considering blocks and barriers,
  (f) assessing support and resistance.
(3) Planning action (equating action with need)
  (a) deciding on the approach to follow,
  (b) identifying resources,
  (c) clarifying the success outcomes needed,
  (d) building the support team,
  (e) securing sanction/political support.

    (4) Taking action (minimal interventions)
- (a) communicating the need for change widely,
- (b) explaining, informing, engaging and supporting,
- (c) taking the minimum change initiative needed,
- (d) allowing for and anticipating problems and unexpected difficulties,
- (e) keeping people involved and informed.

    (5) Sustaining and maintaining (helping continuity)
- (a) considering how to reinforce and sustain the changes,
- (b) involving many in maintaining the new situation,
- (c) ensuring regular review of performance to targets.

This is an outline of the planning framework and the type of questions and considerations to be explored at the various stages in the proess. You will see that the emphasis is heavily in favour of diagnosing the need for change and then planning for action. This covers both *what* needs to be done and *how* best to take action in that particular setting.

Success in implementing change often comes from quality of the diagnosis and planning phases of major change initiatives. Yet often this is not seen or acknowledged. It is of paramount importance however that those doing the diagnosis and planning are closely involved and are not isolated (they need to be field-based generals). They must know what is needed and be skilled in the art of the possible and sustainable. For each of these stages ask yourself what additional points you would ask or want to ensure were given attention. You can build up this framework further to create your own model to use in change management.

Helpful models and ideas

At some stage in your career you will have responsibility for taking forward a change. It may have arisen from an initiative you began or it could be something that you have been asked to do as part of your job. This could be a change to the organization of a clinic or a rescheduling of the duty schedules for a staff group. It could be taking responsibility for the overall management of the ward with a brief to enhance performance.

You have several choices in what to do next with those who will be affected by the changes. You could decide to confront, consult or just act. You could disclose the brief you have been given to make changes, and tell your colleagues what you want done, or you could ask for their ideas about how to proceed. You have many choices open to you. Each one will have certain consequences, both positive and negative. Often there will be some constraints and limiting factors that will influence the choice you make. Factors such as the history of that group, your own management style, how you see yourself and what you assess is the right way forward, will affect your decision about how to proceed.

Whatever you decide, there are some simple and easy-to-use diagnostic models you can use to help you. They can be applied to every change scenario and you can expect them to bring dividends every time. Each can be completed in great detail or they can be used to get a quick overview of the situation in question and then to form the basis for a more extensive diagnosis at some later stage. It is to these we now turn.

The change equation

This is a fundamental building block towards achieving understandable, acceptable, realistic and sustainable change. Using it can alert you to gaps in your thinking about the changes you want to make. It also suggests where you may need to give more effort and attention if you want your proposals to have any chance of success.

The change equation holds that there are three conditions that need to be satisfied if the proposed change is to have a chance of success.

(1) There needs to be sufficient unease with the current situation for those within it to recognize the need for a change.
(2) There has to be sufficient clarity of what and how the future will be different, and beneficial, if a change were made.
(3) Given conditions one and two there has to be some idea of what detailed steps need to be taken to begin moving ahead.

Even if these three conditions are met sufficiently for the proposed change to seem viable, attractive and relevant it then has to be assessed. This needs to take account of the financial, psychological, political etc., costs involved in making the changes before the decision to go ahead can be made.

The change equation is shown in Fig. 13.3. It is a straightforward way of clarifying your thinking. This can be done before you express your

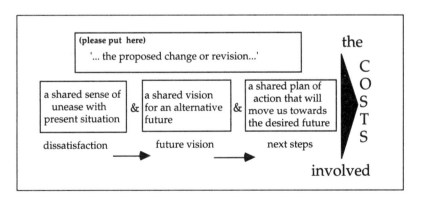

Fig. 13.3 The change equation.

ideas to others. It also helps others to be clearer about their plans and proposals too. You need to check that the effort of changing the *status quo* is worth the costs involved. Costs in terms of money, time, resources, disruption to services etc., but also the psychological costs and implications too.

You will see that I have added in the word *shared* to the three boxes. If you want to implement a successful change you need to bring others with you. Then the sense of dissatisfaction, desired future alternative and how to make a start have to be shared preconditions for successful change.

Note too that each of these three components forms an integral part of the total picture. You could have problems if you try to move ahead without all three of these geared towards change. I have reflected on what it could be like if only one of these three conditions were met, the following scenarios explain the consequences:

(1) *If shared dissatisfaction only:* increasing disappointment with current position and frustration will build up because there is no agreement on what we should have in its place, or understanding of what we should be doing to start making the changes needed.

(2) *If shared vision of the future only:* we can see an alternative to what we have and that looks attractive but there is no reason for us to change. Anyway, even if we wanted to make some changes, we don't know where to start.

(3) *If shared knowledge of first steps only:* we know how we could alter our situation but why should we? It feels comfy, and anyway we don't know yet what we want instead.

Could you speculate what it would be like to be in the situations described in Fig. 13.4? For example case (4). People are dissatisfied with the current position and there is agreement about what they want. Yet there could be extreme frustration because there is no agreed view about what they should *do* to make a start on the change programme. No detailed plan, no sequence of steps to follow. To create this scenario, which could become an increasingly volatile one, would be unwise unless the intention was to create a revolution.

Think about these scenarios and make a note of how you see them. You may find that they describe scenarios already experienced at work. The change equation is a simple way of checking if these three prerequisites for change are in place before any action is initiated.

If the three components are not in place, you could cause confusion and disarray within the organization if you went ahead with some change proposals. This in turn could reduce the morale of staff and affect levels of patient care. It could also bring into disrepute what were appropriate and worthy ideas and proposals for change.

	Shared dis-satisfaction	shared Vision of the future	shared understanding of next steps
Case # 4	present	present	**not present**
Case # 5	present	**not present**	present
Case # 6	**not present**	present	present

Fig. 13.4 Using the change equation to anticipate problems.

Before plans for change are finalized and publicized, it is worth clarifying your thinking by using this approach. It may highlight gaps in your ideas that need to be attended to more fully. It will also help you to plan the sequence of introducing your proposals to others.

Lewin's force field analysis

This is a classic idea of many years standing (Lewin, 1948). I find it as fresh, helpful and as practical as when I first encountered it some time ago. Lewin suggests that every situation we encounter can be looked at as if it were the result of a balance between many conflicting forces and pressures. There will be a range of influences and pressures that want it to alter and another set of forces and influences that want to keep things as they are. The result is a temporary balance creating the seemingly stable situation in front of us. The stability is however an illusion. Far from being fixed, what we see in front of us is a state of balance, a condition of dynamic equilibrium between opposing influences.

If you look at situations – particularly as interpersonal ones in this way – it transforms them. Rather than seeing situations as stable enduring entities, they become recast as flexible and variable.

If you look at relationships and situations as being the result of a balance of opposing influences you can see that the potential for change comes through a realignment of the influences and forces that are in operation. It is the same for organizations. Although on a different scale, organizations develop through a whole range of patterns of influence and history that lead them to their present state. If you change the power, the force or the range of influences and pressures exerted on an organization, then you can change the existing situation.

This method opens up another way of facilitating change in organizations. You can examine a work situation by carefully noting the factors and influences that may be active in creating the situation you are confronting now. By looking at situations as being made up of many 'fields of influence' you have the opportunity to rearrange things and allow change to take place. Figure 13.5 shows the steps involved in building up a force field analysis of your chosen example.

Step 1: WHAT IS THE CHANGE –

Write out clearly *what you are seeking to do* (revise staffing levels; change the system for duty rosters, build better team relationships, stop smoking etc.)

Step 2: SUPPORTING FORCES –

Write out a list of all the influencing factors that *support the change* you want (these can be formal directives, informal things, social pressures, ethical reasons, personal reasons, hidden agendas etc.) – do this as fully as you can.

Step 3: OPPOSING FORCES –

Write out why the change you want is being *opposed* (formal things, assumptions others may be holding, fear and unexpressed worries, personal reasons, loss of power for others, job security fears etc.) – here again as fully as you can.

Step 4: CONTRAST THE DATA –

Put this data together in a way that displays the forces supporting the change wanted against those opposing the desired changes. In this way you can start to build up a concise overview of what seems to you is involved in the matters under review. What this often does is to indicate that (i) there are a great many influencing factors and forces involved, and (ii) that these are operating at several different levels at the same time (e.g. formal, informal, covert, unconscious etc.).

(continued in Fig. 13.7)

Fig. 13.5 Building up a force field.

The format in Fig. 13.6 is often used to contrast the forces *for* change with the forces *against* the change considered. By drawing a force field in this way you get a good sense of the effect these influences have in creating the current *status quo*.

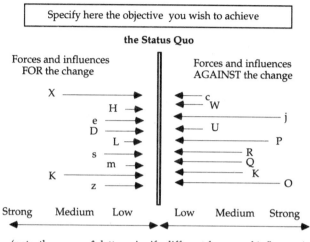

(note: the arrows & letters signify different forces and influences)

Fig. 13.6 An outline force field analysis.

In Fig. 13.6 I have shown several different influences that are affecting the situation I want to change. I have indicated that some of these are exerting a stronger influence than others. At the moment there is a balance achieved between the two sides. This results in the present situation. If I want to alter the current situation I have two basic choices. I can add more power to the forces *for* change side, and/or I can try to reduce the power of the forces *resisting* the proposed changes. Either of these strategies will affect the balance of forces between the two and lead to a new *status quo* (balance point).

The common response to meeting resistance to one's ideas is to restate, even more strongly, the logical and emotional reasons for the change. In other words you try to push it through. This doesn't often work. It can have the annoying effect of causing others to resist what you want even more strongly than before. This makes the situation even more difficult to retrieve for the future. I have been in situations where this has resulted in a rapid and dramatic escalation that stopped just short of physical violence. Only by intervention was the heat taken out of the situation.

If you push for what you want, however well argued and supported by your facts, it does not always lead to acceptance. In terms of the force field diagram in Fig. 13.6, it is the equivalent of increasing the power and thrust of one of the forces for change that then has the knock-on effect of resistance. Although it is possibly a defensive response, it can increase the opposing forces against a change and lead to a worse stalemate than before. As the stakes rise (professionally and personally) so the possibility for an easy climb down become more remote.

A force field analysis however prompts you to consider a complementary change strategy. In addition to increasing the 'pushing' forces, a change can also result if the resisting forces are reduced. This, for me, is the real delight of Lewin's idea. That, it is not just about pushing harder for something, it is the idea of (i) understanding the situation more fully and (ii) seeing if some of the resistance and blocks to action can be reduced or even eliminated. This can then lead to a rebalancing of that situation and the opportunity for change to take place.

The skill is to look for the resistance. See why colleagues are feeling that way, and see what can be done to ease their fears or explain the reasons more fully. For example, you may find that considerable anxiety is provoked by your proposals for change. At the heart of these are:

- fears about personal competence in the new situation,
- fear of failure,
- worries about job security and tenure,
- distrust of management (or nurses, doctors, psychologists) etc.

If these fears and anxieties are unfounded then you need to bring these concerns into public debate. You can then inform people about these aspects of the changes proposed and allay their concerns. If this can be achieved you will notice less resistance and the possibility of more interest in the proposals.

It will never be possible to totally remove resistance. However, if you agree with the logic behind Lewin's approach you may only need to reduce two or three of the resisting forces for the needed changes to happen. So with this in mind the next steps are depicted in Fig. 13.7.

The force field is a way of diagnosing a situation, a means of planning for change and a way of implementing a change strategy and programme. Figure 13.8 is an example of a force field to show you how one looks in practice.

By looking at the example in Fig. 13.8, you can judge what influences this person who wants to give up smoking. The key to the change is to assess which of the resisting forces can be reduced or eliminated altogether. Which do you think could be reduced? My thoughts would be:

- 'Something to do',
- 'Want to be different',
- 'Show rebellion'.

Step 5: PLANNING & ORGANISING –

Look at the data you have recorded and put similar items together to make it easier for you to work from after your initial brainstorming in Steps 2 and 3. You will probably see clusters and groups of items that are similar. Add in other items that you have missed initially. You are now in a position to look at the whole picture, as you see it, of what you think is going on in and around the situation you want to change.

Step 6: ACTIONS –

Now look to see which of the resisting forces you think it is possible to reduce, perhaps by explaining your proposals more carefully, by allaying redundancy fears perhaps, through allowing representation on a change steering group etc. Select three or four of the forces against change that you will start to concentrate on and aim to reduce if possible.

Decide if there is an optimum sequence – for example explain the proposals more fully first, then offer a place on the change steering group etc. – and if so follow it.

Fig. 13.7 A continuation of Fig. 13.5.

See if there are other ways in which this person could be different, show their rebellion and non-conformity. If they have more to do this could make the change easier to accomplish. At some stage the addictive aspects will have to be addressed but at the start this would be difficult to tackle. Conversely, there are some influential reasons why the person wants to make this change. Reasons such as disapproval from their partner, medical reasons etc., and pressure to do something might be stepped up on these.

It is a powerful approach to use. You can do it on your own or with a group, perhaps in a case conference, or on a training course as a way of reviewing a situation.

The gap model

The gap model is about setting direction for the future from a firm starting point. You may recall the joke about some tourists in a car who

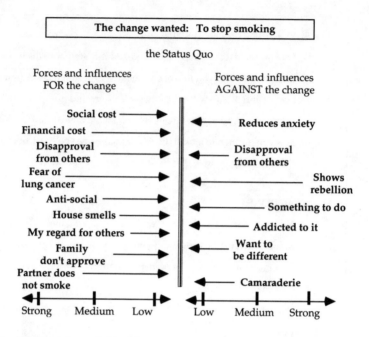

Fig. 13.8 A force field analysis: to stop smoking.

have lost their way. After driving around for some time they decide to ask the way to their desired destination. Eventually they see someone and ask for directions to their destination. The person offers the immortal words: 'Well if I were you I wouldn't start from here...' The same can occur when making changes in organizations. Unless you are clear about where you want to get to and where you are starting from, it is inevitable that you will end up in a place, or in a condition, that you didn't want!

It thus makes sense to:

- be as clear as you can be about the current situation,
- clarify what you want, or need, it to be like in the future.

Then if you have some idea of the difference between now and the future you can:

- get a sense of what effort may be needed for such changes to be accomplished,
- make the changes if they seem viable and realistic.

This can be shown diagrammatically as shown in Fig. 13.9. This simple model compares where you are now with the future situation. This is your *desired* future position that you want to reach in one or two years.

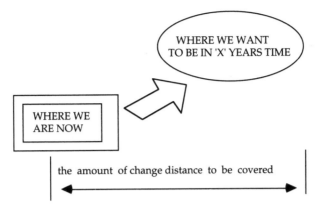

Fig. 13.9 The gap model.

The first step is to list the organizational dimensions that you see need to be developed, introduced etc. Then assess how these are functioning and if there are any problems. So you can complete an assessment of 'Where we are now'.

Step two involves describing as far as you can the desired future position. This focuses on the same functional dimensions you have just described in step one.

Step three involves setting out, as precisely as possible, the major differences between the current and the desired future position. This shows you what the 'gap' is and what will have to be achieved if you are to reach your desired future. It could be that the 'gap' is felt to be too much to attempt or that the organization, department, clinic or teaching department is not yet ready to make a start. But this process concentrates attention on the practicalities of what will be involved. Also the effort and resources needed to achieve the changes desired. Figure 13.10 suggests a format you can use to build up the work into an agenda for change. This will then move you to where you want to be.

By specifying what will need to be altered, introduced as new or maintained as now, focuses the mind on the work required. It could be that as a result of this type of 'gap analysis' the plans for change are put on hold until later.

Symptoms or causes?

When problems arise it is sometimes easier to deal with them immediately. However, sometimes you sense that the problem you have been given is not the real matter that needs the attention.

One of the reasons you may want to change something at work could be because of a difficulty or a problem that recurs frequently. In spite of

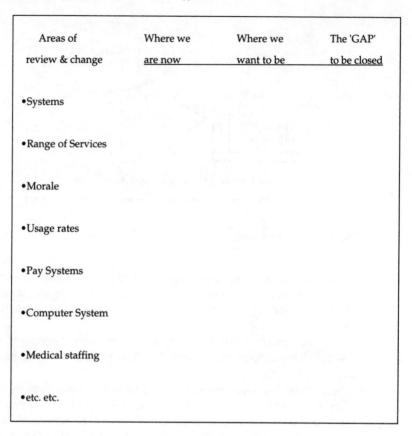

Areas of review & change	Where we are now	Where we want to be	The 'GAP' to be closed
•Systems			
•Range of Services			
•Morale			
•Usage rates			
•Pay Systems			
•Computer System			
•Medical staffing			
•etc. etc.			

Fig. 13.10 Defining the change agenda.

your past action, advice, support etc., you cannot seem to solve the problem. You may think some more decisive action is needed. Or it could be that more *insightful thinking* is needed to determine the problem.

For example, it may be that the problem is not the real issue but is a symptom of something else. If this is the case it would explain why the difficulties have been recurring persistently. Unknown to you, you have been responding to the symptoms and not the causes of the problem.

There are often very good reasons why colleagues don't want to disclose the underlying problem causing them difficulties at work. What reasons do you think these could be? Use Fig. 13.11 to put forward your suggestions (see Fig. 13.15 for some examples). When this happens it does not necessarily mean that a person is being manipulative, secretive, or uncooperative. It is more likely that they are experiencing some pressure. You may be able to relieve some of their stress if you are alert to this possibility rather than only concentrating on work problems.

```
        •

        •

        •

        •
```

Fig. 13.11 Some reasons for not disclosing my underlying problems.

Three examples from my experience are shown in Fig. 13.12. Can you also recall similar examples?

	Presented Problem	**Underlying Difficulty/Problem**
Case 1:	persistent lateness	undisclosed family difficulty
Case 2 :	inaccurate figure taking	break-up with fiancee
Case 3:	recently promoted high-flyer couldn't make simple decisions	fear of failure suddenly overwhelmed everything else

Fig. 13.12 Some examples of undisclosed problems.

In each of these cases there is a presenting problem to which you need to respond. You could respond to what you see in front of you but you may also want to give that person the opportunity to disclose other matters resulting, or contributing, to their work problems.

For example, you could discipline the first two people and tell them to 'pull their socks up'. You could support and encourage the third person and remind them that they are doing an excellent job. In each case you could, unintentionally, make their situation worse. Instead it is important to make it possible for them to talk about their underlying problems. These are the anxieties and pressures causing the symptoms you see at work.

If it does emerge that there are other causal factors then these are the matters that need to be taken in hand. If the distress they are causing can be reduced, there will be less reason for the symptoms you see at work to persist. You must also be aware that, as their boss, you may not be the best person to work through such personal and private material. This is because it may confuse and complicate the work relationship between the two of you. This is not to say that problems cannot be shared or talked about. However, when a deeper exploration of what is on their mind is required, occupational health, or counselling support services are the appropriate people to be involved, if the person agrees.

It is like the analogy of the iceberg. What you actually see from the surface is only the small part above the waterline. Underneath is a huge mass that is not seen. It is the same with symptoms and causes. We see the symptoms but they are not necessarily what we need to be looking at. It is what is causing them in the first place – as Fig. 13.13 illustrates – that needs to be attended to.

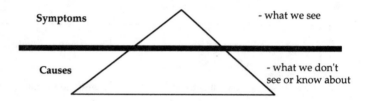

Fig. 13.13   Symptoms and underlying causes.

The representation of a person's concerns as symptoms, rather than their underlying cause, often indicates that the person is not ready or in a position to show the causal issue and concern. Therefore you need to take great care in finding out if there is something else driving their symptoms. You may not be the most appropriate person to become involved in such explorations. However, you do have a role to seek why the difficulties are there and if there are other concerns causing them.

Make or break: the key influencers

In most situations there are just a few people whose support is needed for your ideas for change to have a chance of success. There are also only a few of those whose opposition could render your plans unacceptable. Securing such support is a vital objective. This small group of key influencers are often called 'the critical mass'. You need to get as many of them on your side as you can.

The first step is to decide who they are. Make a list of those people whom you see to be the critical ones, in relation to the specific changes you are suggesting. The next step is to summarize individually the degree of support they have for your ideas. Figure 13.14 shows one way of doing this.

In this example there are 11 people whose commitment is very important for the change to take place. Of these I assess that the majority will either help and support me or don't see the changes as a

The key people	Will make	Will stop	Will help	Will allow	Don't care
Sister X	■				
Sister XX		■			
Dr Z				■	
Dr F					■
Mr K			■		
Nurse S			■		
C/N B	■				
Business Manager	■				
Clinical Director		■			
Pathology					■
Ward Manager	■				

Fig. 13.14   Charting the critical mass.

matter of concern to them. But I do have a problem with the clinical director and with Sister XX. Their support is very necessary for the new arrangements to work successfully.

I will need to understand more fully why they don't want the changes to go ahead and to see if I can allay their reservations and doubts. At the very least I need to see if I can move them from a position of opposition to one which allows the changes to go ahead.

The fact that I have located the business manager in the 'will make' it happen column shows she shares my view of the need for change. The ward manager is on board as well as very positive. It is unfortunate that some of the care team seem not to care at all but at least they will not disrupt or block the change if it goes ahead.

Now, this is only my view and like everyone else my views are biased. Thus it can be very helpful for my perspectives to be checked by colleagues working with me on this change. After we have agreed who we see as the critical people, we can independently complete the chart in Fig. 13.14 and compare notes. Often there are differences and these can then be worked through to consider how we can best approach those we see as blocking the work planned and to address the difficulties they are suggesting.

Chapter 14 now considers the role of the nurse as a facilitator of change. This is often referred to as a 'change agent'.

Worked example

- embarrassed

- don't feel confidentiality will be maintained

- I will be judged as week and wimpish

- no understanding will be forthcoming

- I don't know what the problem is

- fear of ....

Fig. 13.15   Some reasons for not disclosing my underlying problems.

Reference

Lewin, K. (1948) *Resolving Social Conflicts*, Harper, New York.

Further reading

Beckhard, R. and Harris, R. (1987) *Organizational Transitions* (2nd edn), Addison-Wesley, Reading, MA.

Brunning, H., Cole, C. and Huffington, C. (1990) *The Change Directory*, British Psychological Society, Leicester.

Carter, R. *et al.* (1984) *Systems, Management and Change*, Harper and Row, London.

McCalman, J. and Paton, R. (1992) *Change Management*, Paul Chapman, London.

Spurgeon, P. and Barwell, F. (1991) *Implementing Change in the NHS*, Chapman and Hall, London.

Chapter 14
The Nurse as Change Agent and Facilitator

Of all the professionals who provide care and attention the nursing function is the one which is always present on the ward. In clinics and on home and community visits it will generally be the nurses who occupy the most prominent and continuing of the care roles provided. When asked who they see most of, and who they view as their primary carer it will probably be the nurse(s) who comes most readily to the patient's mind.

The nurse's role continually reviews and monitors a patient's well-being. More than any other professional they are able to assess the state of play of their patients and provide overall assessments about the ward, clinic, etc. Of all the care providers nurses have the most extensive network of 'ground' intelligence. They know what is going on, where difficulties arise, what needs attention and support and – critically – what needs to be re-examined and perhaps changed.

This highlights the role of the nurse as a force for change and review, based on the practical realities of care delivery. Often before any other staff, nurses will have a shrewd idea of what will work and are a valuable source of information about the organization, its procedures and its performance. Nurses are 'agents of change' in addition to their professional direct-care provider role.

The nurse:

- has continuity of patient contact,
- has a formalized, detailed and regular updating system in place,
- is often the 'most seen' member of the caring team,
- is the regular point of contact for the wider care support team, relatives, etc.,
- has 24 hour coverage of the hospital.

The nurse is at the heart of the care network for the patients under her care. She can assess the mood of the hospital throughout the day. It is like being at the centre of an information and decision-making web. The person (or people) at the centre are well placed to make sense of, and integrate, all the data available. They are the best placed to assess, at any one time, the needs and demands of the patient, and perhaps, also for parts of the organization itself.

The nurse is in a central position from which to influence, oversee and manage the implementation of decisions about patient care strategies. She can also facilitate changes to ward or clinic administrative practices. The training of the nurse provides a sound grounding to cope with and facilitate personal change and adaptation. These are skills fundamental to successful work as a change facilitator.

The responsibilities of the nurse on the ward or in the clinic may not allow time for change facilitation work beyond patient care. Yet it is through this period that the nurse will be learning and practising her change skills. This is not to say that every nurse will want to develop further this part of her role but some of the key change facilitation skills and attributes needed for successful change agents will have been developed. Figure 14.1 lists some of the key characteristics for success in facilitating change. To what extent do you match these?

• seen as competent	• successful professional track record
• respected professional	• takes a broad organisational perspective
• thoughtful & considered	• has experience on the ground
• politically astute	• understands the positions of others
• communicates clearly	• works through opinion leaders
• seen as credible	• has business diagnostic skills
• open to review ideas	• able to engage others
• politically informed	• offers support/development to client
• ethically straightforward	• can visualise future states
• seen to 'care' for people and the organisation	
• aware of own strengths and weaknesses	

Fig. 14.1   Key characteristics in facilitating change.

From my experience the essential characteristics of component and well respected change agents are:

- good diagnostic skills,
- sound theoretical knowledge of this field,
- an ability to relate well to others and 'see' things from the client's perspective,
- internal political awareness and sensitivity,
- personal integrity and clarity of purpose,

- an ability to take care of others,
- a willingness to take care of themself,
- an ability to communicate and be heard at all levels,
- a 'supervisor' to talk with about change problems.

If you look at these abilities and attributes they are precisely the kind of abilities we all need to get on in the world. They are not overly technical, and do not require years of dedicated study. They are the 'life and living skills' that we have all developed to varying degrees over the years. Sometimes our ability to exercise them may have been impeded by unhelpful experiences along the way. But life skills are meant to be honed and developed through reflections on our experiences and what we have observed in others.

If you agree with this assessment, it follows that each of us is a facilitator, or has the potential to be one. An interesting proposition don't you think? It also follows that each of us has the potential to alter, make sense of and develop the situations in which we find ourselves. Because of your training and experience with patients over protracted periods of time you already have considerable insight into human nature and what helps and hinders change.

Purposes of a change agent

You know from experience though that just because a person has potential for something it does not follow that they will necessarily want to exercise or develop that capability further. It is the same with these abilities. There is great strain – intellectual and emotional – involved in facilitating more effective working relationships and change. Not everyone wants that responsibility.

If you are a change agent you seek to do the following:

- to facilitate constructive review and change,
- to draw relevant matters into discussion,
- to create possibilities for development.

While these statements may look straightforward, they are difficult to achieve and require considerable skills and personal awareness. However, the diagnostic and change capabilities, if suitably developed, can be applied irrespective of a person's formal job title, or role.

While your formal role may limit or constrain the scope you have to fully develop some of the above attributes, it need not stop you from:

- noticing what is going on around you,
- trying to make sense of it,
- monitoring your own and the changing reactions of those around you.

Because of the role you occupy you have affect and can influence what goes on around you. To do so with success and care you need to have a way of structuring your activities and of knowing how to improve your skills and knowledge. Figure 14.2 suggests four core change agent roles each of which requires an array of skills and abilities.

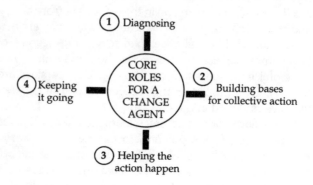

Fig. 14.2   Core change agent skills.

The nurse, in a change facilitation role, is seen by those affected by the proposed changes as a relevant and acceptable person. They are likely to be content that she is involved and will work with them in helping change happen. So the nurse as 'change agent' is often able to be allowed in, to *gain entry* to the client situation and has *credibility* in such a role in the eyes of those involved. These two matters are critically important because unless they are secured whatever work you try to do will be flawed and, at some point, could fail.

Figure 14.2 suggests four key roles (and phases) in the process of facilitating review and change. I deliberately use the word review because you may find that there is no need for change after you have diagnosed the client situation.

The first, and critical stage is about *diagnosing* what is going on and in understanding how things function. The second major stage is about *building shared understandings* of the need for action. Also for some agreement on what is wanted in place of the current arrangements. The third stage is about *helping the changes happen*. If things run smoothly and succeed there should be no surprise experienced by those affected. The fourth stage is about *keeping it going; securing the positive benefits* from the changes and maintaining them over time.

Figure 14.3 notes some of the tasks that need to be covered at each of these stages and some of the skills and attributes required.

I have suggested that each of us has the potential to function in a facilitative way at work. Yet not everyone welcomes or values the possible change agent roles outlined. There are personal costs associated with helping constructive change happen. You know from your

Main Tasks to undertake	Skills & Knowledge needed
DIAGNOSIS	
Finding out and collecting data (listening, watching, asking), speculating, Diagnosing the need for review/change	Ability to relate well to others at all levels; intellectually bright and astute, attentive listening etc.
BUILDING SHARED BASE FOR ACTION	
Building the base for change (mobilising understandings and support)	Presenting a sound and robust case, sensitivity to the needs of others, able to tolerate challenge, emotionally strong. Competent strategic and tactical thinker
TAKING ACTION	
Supporting and encouraging relevant actions that enable the client system to address its issues	Resolute and determined in aiding client, builds competence and confidence in client system
KEEPING IT GOING	
Maintaining and sustaining the changes - helping them to bed-down successfully	Providing support and continuity of care

Fig. 14.3 Summary of core change agent roles.

experiences of intervening in situations how those to whom you were offering support can, on occasion, suddenly turn on you, or whilst you thought you were doing a good piece of work you suddenly realize with horror that it is all going wrong and out of control.

There is a high emotional price to be paid and considerable intellectual application is needed to function with sensitivity and success as a change agent. It may also become apparent that others begin to stereotype you when you are working in this way and begin to hold unrealistic expectations of what you can do and what you can deliver.

Stereotypes of change agents

Given the material we have covered in Part Four how would you stereotype a person who is a facilitator of changes in the workplace? You will recall that we can hold unrealistic expectations of, or even fantasies about, those who exercise significant influence on us at work (see Part Two).

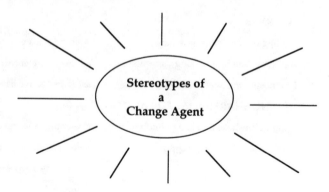

Fig. 14.4   Stereotypes of a change agent: Part 1.

When you complete Fig. 14.4, be as frank as you can. You can even exaggerate because by clarifying what the extreme stereotypes may be we can be clearer about what is really on the minds of those holding the stereotypes. Figure 14.5 shows some of my thoughts drawn from material I have read and written over the years about this type of work. No doubt you may have other images that occur to you. What do you do if these are the sort of feelings, images, and expectations that colleagues have when 'change agent' (or facilitator, or consultant etc.) is mentioned? How will these thoughts affect their work relationship with you?

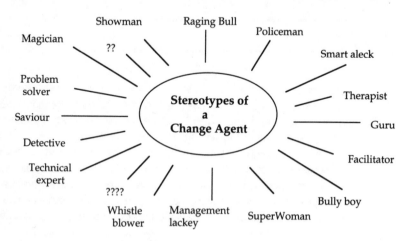

Fig. 14.5   Stereotypes of a change agent: Part 2.

One strategy is to explain more carefully what the role of facilitating internal change means. Another possibility is to show colleagues different ways of diagnosing and describing organizational situations. In this way you build up their understanding of the type of work involved. Your aim is to dispel some of the unrealistic and counter-productive stereotypes noted in Fig. 14.5. Your aim is to establish the work of a change agent on a realistic level.

The most critical question about helping change happen revolves around why you would want to do this in the first place. I have no doubt that the nurse is well placed to influence and affect many things. She can make things go smoothly and has a store of detailed local knowledge that can be applied positively, if she chooses. Knowing why you want to exercise your change agent potential will help you manage the stresses and pleasures such work generates.

It is worth asking yourself the following questions:

- Who are you doing it for?
- What are your motivations and interests?
- Who is the client?
- What do you want out of it?
- Is it worth it and how will you assess this?

I believe these roles are immensely important in helping organizations function as smoothly as possible. I think also there can be considerable pressure placed on change agents (some of it self-induced!) to solve the problems and issues identified. By being clearer about your role you will be helped to maintain an overall perspective. It will also help you to understand a little more about why this type of work matters to you.

Being described as a 'change agent' can be appealing and it has a glamour associated with it. What is often not recognized is the careful attention needed to use the type of models set out in Chapter 13 and the various attributes noted earlier in this chapter.

Most of this book has been about trying to understand yourself, about others and about organizations and then deciding if anything needs to change. There will be some things you now want to change and Part Four has looked at the difficulties involved from an organization development perspective.

Further reading

Argyris, C. (1970) *Intervention Theory and Method*, Addison-Wesley, Reading, MA.

Argyris, C. (1990) *Overcoming Organizational Defences*, Allyn and Bacon, Boston, MA.

Blake, R. and Mouton, J. (1976) *Consultation*, Addison-Wesley, Reading, MA.

Block, P. (1981) *Flawless Consulting*, Learning Concepts, Austin, Texas.

Brunning, H. *et al.* (1990) *The Change Directory*, British Psychological Society, Leicester.

Lippitt, G. and Lippitt, R. (1978) *The Consulting Process in Action*, University Associates, La Jolla, CA.

McCalman, J. and Paton, R. (1992) *Change Management*, Paul Chapman Publishing, London.

Ridgeway, C. and Wallace, B. (1994) *Empowering People*, Institute of Personnel and Development, London.

Steele, F. (1975) *Consulting for Organizational Change*, University of Massachusetts Press, Amherst, MA.

PART FIVE:
WORKING IN THE PRESSURE COOKER

It is very easy to become so interested by the detail that the broader context is forgotten. Chapters 15 and 16 re-emphasize the health care contexts you work in. They also re-emphasize the book's purpose in encouraging you to build up a clearer sense of who you are as a person and as a carer.

I hope you have been interested and intrigued by the various chapters. The optimum benefits will come if you can integrate all these ideas and perspectives together and use them appropriately where you work. While the early chapters are valuable in themselves it is when you use them together that you are most likely to generate new and constructive approaches to current problems and difficulties.

In thinking about the changing NHS, the changing nursing role and the very publicized debates on health care, it seems to me that it is like working in a pressure cooker. This book suggests ways in which you may be able to sustain that pressure, provide good care, support colleagues and look after yourself in the process.

Chapter 15
Back to the Organization

Although you have been appointed to fulfil certain tasks your ability to do this is constrained by the organization you work in. You may be the brightest in your year, the youngest nurse specialist ever appointed in your hospital, etc. However, how you deliver care is tied up with wider matters than solely your professional energy, insight, competence and commitment. If this is so you need to decide how best you can function and work productively within organizations. I often hear of professionals giving up because of frustration with 'the system'. This may be accurate yet often it is that they themselves have not been able to work well enough within the constraints around them.

You are very unlikely to be given a totally free hand in the work you do. There will always be constraints and limitations that get in the way. Thus it may be more productive to think of *how* to work within such constraints rather than against them. I am not advocating inaction – where there are major problems – or complacency. Clearly if there is a major problem, or operational dysfunction, these will need to be resolved but I am thinking of the local ways of doing things that you may find irksome and would not normally follow if you were given a free hand.

Part One touched on the history of health care in the UK and on some aspects of organizational life. You know that the culture of your organization developed over the years will influence how things are done and that it is very difficult to alter the *status quo*. The style of the chief executive, the chairperson, the key clinicians etc., also exerts tremendous influence on what occurs in the trust, clinic and so on. You know also that external influences can challenge and change the whole structure of care provision. They can affect what, and how, you want to function as a professional.

Figure 15.1 is a reminder of the demands and sources of pressure which you are trying to balance, make sense of and feel comfortable with, as you go about your work.

Each of these 'constituencies' exert an influence on you to conform to their needs. They constrain and limit your actions and your thinking. When you work inside an organization there are pressures put on you to conform to its way of doing things. In return benefits such as security,

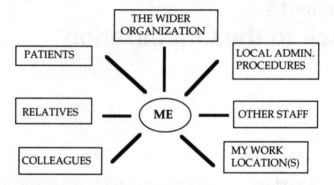

Fig. 15.1 Sources of influence acting on me.

mutual support, group cohesion, prospects, professional status and protection are offered. Being part of an organization differentiates you, and your colleagues, from others who are not part of that 'community' but this places expectations on you and imposes restrictions. Figure 15.1 reminds you of some of the sources of these confirmatory and restrictive pressures and pulls.

To remain effective it is necessary to keep these constraints in mind. You need to decide, while remaining ethical, caring and pragmatic, how to work within these constraints. If appropriate, you could help them to be reviewed and changed.

As a nurse in an organization many demands are placed on you over and above providing direct patient care. Yet these additional expectations, stresses and pressures can easily be forgotten, and their impact discounted. If you think about the range of pressures on you (excluding those to do with patient treatment) what would they be? I have put down a few initial thoughts in Fig. 15.2.

These two figures highlight the many considerations and pressures that will affect the delivery of your professional skills to your patients. To remain fully effective in a health care organization requires you to come to terms with these pressures. These are in addition to those that arise from your clinical work. One way you can do this is to build up a picture of where you work now. This could be similar to Fig. 15.1 and show the main influences and dynamics that are in force. Then when issues arise you will be more able to:

- identify where they are coming from,
- be able to make more sense of them as part of the broader perspective on the organization, and its workings, than if you only saw things from solely a ward perspective,
- put them into perspective,
- deal with them in a more informed manner,

- think which aspects of the broader picture you want to change and in what way,
- build up your own change agenda,
- start developing your own change strategy.

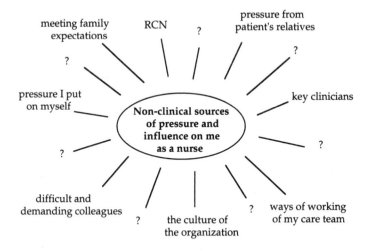

Fig. 15.2 Non-clinical pressures on me.

If you don't have a broader view in mind it will be harder to cope with the pressures you experience and you may increasingly begin to feel that the job is getting you down and that you are slowly being pulled apart. Most of us are prone to see things from a parochial perspective and are liable to miss the bigger picture and opportunities to influence and change things.

When you say 'organization', which one do you mean?

When you build up a 'picture' of your organization, remember that there is more than one organization in operation in your trust, DMU or group practice. You need to be clear about what these are and what they mean in practice. This is an important part of 'getting to grips' with what it means to work where you are. However, if you don't know what to start looking for it is unlikely you will find anything unexpected so, set out below are some alternative ways of describing your organization:

- the organization as set out on the formal organization chart,
- the organization as it actually works,
- the organization as its members would like it to be,
- the organization as denied by its members,

- the organization as myth,
- the organization we publicize ourselves to be.

These provide clues about what to look for.

Some of these perspectives are a far cry from the rather classical ideas of formal organizations. Which are seen as operating in a very hierarchical, top-down and linear manner (as in the traditional organization charts). Where there is a job to do and people to do it without deviation or questioning.

Each of these different perspectives about organizations noted above are important to consider. Each exercises an influence on what, and how, things happen. If you look at where you work through these perspectives different things come to prominence. Additional insights emerge that can help to explain more fully what is going on. *What* you look at is still the same. It is *how* you look at it that makes the difference.

To make change, exercise your skills to the full, weather the stresses and strains, and remain effective means you need to know:

- where you are – professionally, and organizationally,
- who you are – psychologically, emotionally and spiritually.

These are difficult and personal matters to consider. One way to begin putting all of these thoughts together is to build up your own maps and frameworks to reflect where you are and what matters to you. During the course of the book you have been asked to reflect, and make notes, on different aspects of yourself and on what you have seen and experienced. As a first step in building up your own frameworks about yourself, you could bring these notes together and integrate them. You could build up a picture of where you work using ideas and frameworks from Parts One, Three and Four which will give you a good idea of what is going on in your workplace. In these ways you can be much clearer about who you are and about the contexts within which you are working.

Chapter 16
Looking after Yourself

This book offers you ways of assessing, and then coping with, the pressures and tensions you experience at work. The person I have kept in mind in writing the book has been a carer – specifically a nurse – working in a health care organization. However, the material could equally be relevant to other health care staff and other work locations.

There are four aims in this book:

(1) For the reader to be more aware of themselves and about some of their own personal issues,
(2) To enable the reader to use ideas, frameworks and models to assess the operational effectiveness of their organization,
(3) For the reader to stimulate constructive change where needed,
(4) To enhance the quality of patient care

I believe that health care professionals, perhaps more than any other of the caring and emergency services, have to endure and cope with intense emotional pressure over prolonged periods. This generates considerable strain. Strain which is all too often glossed over, or discounted, as 'part of the job'. I don't believe this does credit to the tenacity and commitment shown by carers.

This book describes ways of working through some of these tensions and pressures. This can be achieved through the process of clarifying what may be going on and deciding what you can (and want to) do about it. The material gives you more control over how you handle the situations you experience. A further step could be for you to discuss those ideas you have found most helpful with your colleagues so that they may also begin to influence and shape things which hitherto they may have taken for granted.

The individuality of the nurse at work – as a person in their own right – is often neglected. This is also true for the emotional impact and strain of being on the ward, in the unit or out in the community. Conventionally rather more attention is given to the other three segments that make up Fig. 16.1 (see also Preface). I suspect this is partly because they are easier to deal with (e.g. the facts, figures, organization charts and job descriptions, etc.). Also it could be partly as a defence against acknowledging the intensity of the emotional pressures nurses experience.

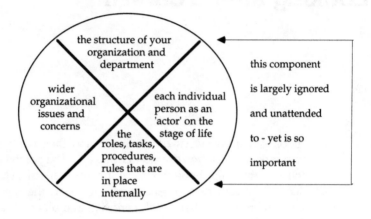

the structure of your
organization and
department

this component

is largely ignored

wider
organizational
issues and
concerns

each individual
person as an
'actor' on the
stage of life

and unattended

to - yet is so

the
roles, tasks,
procedures,
rules that are
in place
internally

important

Fig. 16.1 What gets the attention at work.

Yet it is this personal approach in each of us, while working professional and ethically, that the patient ultimately turns to as a touchstone for the quality of care they are receiving. That is why this book puts you as a person at the heart of the nursing role rather than you as a technical professional.

The book encourages you to build up your knowledge of yourself. So much rests on this and the more you can understand and appreciate yourself – strengths and failings – the more you will be able to care for those around you. Without a sufficient sense of self you may find that you react or try to influence or work in ways that are detrimental to yourself, your patients and others. Remember I am *not* talking about clinical medical care but of how you act, and relate to others, as a person.

The more you are at ease with yourself the more able you will be to make quality caring relationships with your patients, and others and the more you will be able to sustain and put into perspective the psychological stresses and pressures of being a nurse.

The intensity of the issues you encounter at work trigger the full range of human emotions. The professional care you provide leads to a privileged intimacy with a patient that is normally reserved for close family and loved ones. From the start you are very important to your patient and this puts pressure on you. In health care settings your everyday actions can become amplified. The inherent stress and worry that surrounds them can be interpreted by patients (and carers for that matter) to contain more significance and meaning than really exists or was intended.

For patient and carer alike it can seem as if you are living in a goldfish bowl, under the inquisitive view of others. Magnified through the intense attention of observers, the nurse and other care staff can become 'larger than life'. They will be expected by some to be all-knowing and all powerful as previously discussed in Part Three.

It can be likened to working in a pressure cooker. You find that, coming on duty, the heat is turned on and the pressure builds during the day (or night). Consequently, avoid getting too pressured, you need all your resolve to stay intact and operate effectively despite the pressure. Unless you can cope with increasing emotional pressure, moderated by you and your insights, you may try to match the unrealistic expectations of others. Ultimately an impossible venture and one destined for failure and disappointment.

Some thoughts and considerations

To have the best chance of influencing things and moderating the pressures, remember to use some of the material from Part Four. Your plans and proposals must:

- be feasible,
- be understandable to those affected,
- take account of the feelings of those affected,
- be politically acceptable,
- have clear outcomes and benefits,
- be administratively acceptable and convenient.

To be effective, decisions must address the important issues as seen by those affected and be capable of being put into practice both organizationally and personally. However, even your best thought out efforts may not proceed as planned. You may find Fig. 16.2 contains some useful reminders. You can add more of your own.

You can use your completed version of this diagram to remind you that no one can totally cover or manage to control all the variables in any interactional situation. Inevitably there will be outcomes that are unexpected. Not all things will go as planned. Others will work so well that you feel elated for days. The diagram can remind you that try as you may you cannot get it right all of the time. It keeps the reality of life firmly in the foreground.

Taking action

This book offers you a means to build up your personal understandings about the importance of being here, as a person and specifically working as a nurse. This has several benefits, for example:

- to help you to learn more from your experiences,
- to become better prepared for the future,

- to monitor your own feelings and performance,
- to be a little clearer about how you feel about your position.

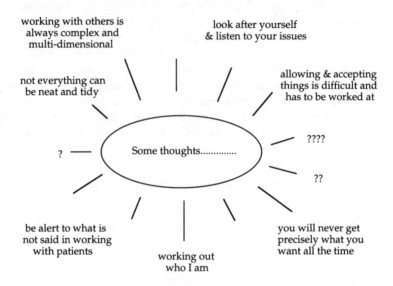

working with others is
always complex and
multi-dimensional

look after yourself
& listen to your issues

not everything can
be neat and tidy

allowing & accepting
things is difficult and
has to be worked at

? —— Some thoughts..............

????

??

be alert to what is
not said in working
with patients

working out
who I am

you will never get
precisely what you
want all the time

Fig. 16.2 Some thoughts and considerations . . .

You will want to add other points to these. However, I expect that since you have been using the ideas and frameworks you will have some idea of which ones have worked well for you. If you are using ideas and approaches that are new to you, don't be disappointed if things don't go according to plan. Building up familiarity with new concepts takes time along with putting them into practice. Persevere and these ideas and approaches will serve you well over many years. This is especially so if you adapt them and make them your own. You may also like to get into the habit of making a regular summary of how things are going for you along the lines of Fig. 16.3.

My hope is that you will use the ideas and models regularly because with more experience of using them you will be able to identify additional dimensions and material to explore.

I hope too that you will be prepared to keep an open mind to new experiences. Avoid, to some extent at least, the following examples noted by Sutherland (1992) of how:

> . . . The reluctance to relinquish one's own views permeates all life. It makes doctors fail to change their diagnoses even when they are clearly wrong; it results in gross injustice . . . ; it makes scientists stick to the theories that have been demonstrably falsified . . . there is often a determination to stick to one's beliefs regardless of the evidence, this tendency is so pervasive that it can affect the way we see or hear.

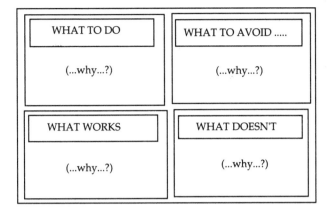

Fig. 16.3 Check how things are going for me, now...

As Sutherland notes, we can be intensely committed and locked into things to such an extent that we lose our perspective and understanding of what is tangible and real. Each of us experiences life differently, we put different emphases on different things and we create our own unique world in the process. Some of this we reveal, and some of it can be discerned by those around us. Some of it we keep inside, and some part of each of us is unknown, even to ourselves. This is even though it influences who we are, what we do and our very being.

This book suggests ways of enabling you to be a little clearer about who you are and how you can work more sensitively with yourself and with others. Take care.

Reference

Sutherland, S. (1992) *Irrationality: The Enemy Within*, Constable, London.

Index